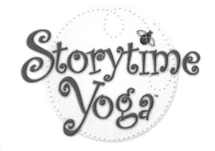

Storytime Yoga

The Treasure in Your Heart

Stories and Yoga
for Peaceful Children

By Sydney Solis
RYT

Edited by
Melanie Sumner

Photographs by
Michelle Maloy Dillon

The Mythic Yoga Studio
Boulder, Colorado

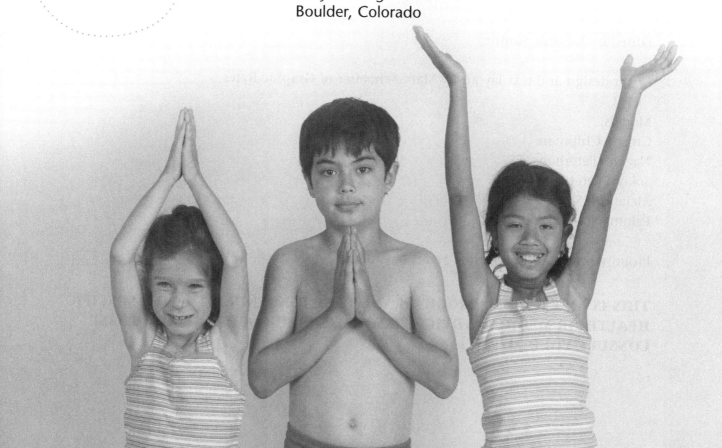

The Mythic Yoga Studio, LLC
PO Box 3805
Boulder, CO 80307

First Edition - Second Printing

Library of Congress Cataloging-In-Publication Data

Library of Congress Control Number: 2007904776

Solis, Sydney, 1966-
Storytime Yoga™: The Treasure in Your Heart – Yoga and Stories for Peaceful Children / by Sydney Solis

ISBN 9780977706310

1. Hatha yoga, for children 2. Exercise, for children 3. Storytelling

To order additional copies of this book, visit www.StorytimeYoga.com.

Photographs by Michelle Maloy Dillon

Edited by Melanie Sumner

Cover design and text layout by Mary Schaeffer of Graphic Bytes

Models:
Crosby Chipman
Nayana Peterhans
Soklyn Peterhans
Alejandro Solis
Paloma Solis

Proudly printed in the United States of America.

THIS IS AN EXERCISE PROGRAM AND IS NOT INTENDED TO GIVE SPECIFIC HEALTH OR MEDICAL ADVICE. BEFORE STARTING A PRACTICE, PLEASE CONSULT YOUR PHYSICIAN

DEDICATED TO

My Mother
Agnes Clara Ann Tichacek Straub
June 10, 1931 – Oct. 11, 2001

And my Father
Albert Edward Louis Straub
May 1, 1933 –

And to my beloved
Justin, Walker, Crosby, Alejandro, and Paloma

Be Noble for You are Made of Earth

Be Humble for You are Made of Stars

~ Serbian Proverb

Acknowledgements

Many heartfelt thanks to the following lights in my life: the children at Creekside and Columbine Elementary Schools in Boulder, Colorado; Louann Harlow of Boulder Parks and Recreation and all the children and families who took classes there; Sherry Patterson, Kathy Ireland and Deborah Cortez of Lakewood Head Start; Aliza Sodos of Littleton Yoga Center; and Andi Johnson of Yoga Elements in Louisville, Colorado.

Thanks to Francie Halderman, Greg Shaw, Gerald McDermott and Bob Walters of the Joseph Campbell Foundation. To Jan Manzer of the Joseph Campbell Foundation Colorado Roundtable for his undying enthusiasm, and to Germaine Dietsch and Bev and Tom Brayden of Spellbinders.

To Melanie Sumner for her friendship and editing and literary expertise and for sending along Pam Redden to edit and proofread. To Susan Kaplan for her friendship, love, peace, kindness and brilliance. To Carole Heepke of the Boulder Public Library for friendship, stories, and community. Thanks to Chuck Hunker and Mark LeBlanc for sensational business coaching and to my assistant Heather Fontenot.

Extra special thanks to Laura Simms and Dan Hessey, as well as Debbie Huttner of the Wellness Initiative, Boulder, Colorado. Also to to Andria Pizzato, Brenda Abdilla, Elizabeth Padilla and Mary Schaeffer.

To Margot Dengel for her undying enthusiasm as a Storytime Yoga™ teacher and to all the Storytime Yoga™ teachers in the League of Yogic Storytellers. You make my heart sing.

To Jeanie Straub of the Parker, Colorado public library for her expertise and brilliance.

And most of all to my beloved Justin Chipman, healer and husband extraordinaire.

I am also extremely grateful for all the suffering I have been given to endure, for this obstacle was indeed the path.

Sydney

Table of Contents

Forward ~ by Laura Simms

Some years ago, as a storyteller/facilitator in a conference called Young Voices at the UN, a girl from Bosnia was asked by a journalist if she knew the causes of war. She answered cheerfully, "I am interested in the causes of peace." She had lived through unimaginable horrors and understood, as did all the young people in that gathering, that there is no winner in war. There is only violence and loss. A book that offers us activities - a means - to uncover, awaken, and joyfully support the inner goodness and capacity for peace in our children is a weapon worth wielding.

Sydney's lovely book of philosophy, heart-motivated activities and inspiring stories with yoga poses is a treasure of clues and inspirations. It offers a practical way to deepen body knowledge and ear to spirit enjoyment for the benefit of children. The book promotes and instigates the enlivening of the causes of peace. The inner spiritual life of children is often ignored, or assumed because it is natural, to be active. However, the muscles of inner relaxation, patience, confidence in one's goodness, resilience and capacity for compassion albeit inherent, need exercise in order to gain strength and flower. We need to learn how to provide our children and ourselves with the zeal for wholesome compassionate living.

I first met Sydney Solis when she took a workshop I was giving at Naropa University. Her immense generosity of listening and unquenchable interest in the power of stories to heal made us fast friends. At the time she was seeking her own way through the dark forest of trauma recovery. She was fresh from the devastating pain of her husband's suicide and her children's confusion. She was reviewing her life with a dedicated looking glass to better understand what had happened. A few years later, engaged in a week-long storytelling residency, it was evident she had transformed her own obstacles into medicine for self and others. She had begun teaching yoga and working with children. Sydney came to study again, but this time to better understand how to help others. I loved each time she got up to tell a story, or to dialogue with students. I savored the trust I felt in her awareness and selfless quest to be the best storyteller possible.

Her storytelling and yoga practice is nurtured by study, experience and courage. To hear Syd tell stories, or to close one's eyes and rest in a pose as she guides us back home to presence, to open heart, to deep wide breathing, is to receive the gift of the healer who has healed herself. This book is filled with profound ideas, and useful tips all based on personal time-tested journeys she has made with children who were lucky enough to have her as a storytelling yoga teacher.

The more that we trust that our children can flourish through listening, breathing, resting the mind, learning the joy of caring for others, and relishing the playful victory of relaxation in their own bodies, regardless of circumstances, the more we are promoting peace in our troubled world. Not only has Syd helped us to remember to look within in order to transform the world, but has beautifully dared to give us a means of uncovering the sources of peace and happiness with our children who are inheriting our world.

Bravo.

Laura Simms

Introduction

On the first day of a six-week after-school yoga class, I ask the children questions about themselves: "Why are you here? What do you know about yoga? What's going on in your life?" Their responses range from "My mom made me do it" to "Yoga is fun" to "School is hard; I need help dealing with stress."

"How are things at home?" I ask.

"Rough," said a little boy named Brian, with a distant look in his eyes. In an instant, I saw myself in him. As I recalled my own childhood, my heart went out to him.

I grew up outside of Boulder, Colorado, in the early 70s. My mother, who was diagnosed with a severe mental illness, physically and verbally abused my three siblings and me. At times, she was creative and joyous: writing poetry, dancing to Eartha Kitt, sewing aprons and placemats to earn an extra buck; but she lived at the mercy of her disease. Sometimes she felt compelled to wake us in the middle of the night, waving a pair of scissors and screaming that she would cut off our hair. Although my father worked hard and made a decent salary, my mother imagined us poor, and we lived in filth and squalor. On the occasions when she suddenly demanded we clean the kitchen floor, we had to get on our knees to scrape up the black goop that came off in curls on our putty knives. My Dutch father, a child-survivor of a Japanese concentration camp on Java during World War II, suffered from a post-traumatic stress disorder that included intense migraine headaches. Most of the time, he acquiesced to my mother.

My mother dressed like a bag lady, shopping for our clothes at garage sales and sometimes digging through the neighbors' garbage cans. While my classmates sported the new Izod shirts with alligators over their hearts, I wore a grease stain that my mother had embroidered over with yellow yarn to disguise its second-hand flaw. But I knew it was there.

As the kids at school and in the neighborhood teased me mercilessly about my clothing and my "weird" mother, I withdrew into a shell of sorrow, anger, and self-hatred. The war within me reflected the sad, confused world around me, and I retreated to a sanctuary of books, stories, and eventually, yoga.

When my father told me a story about his encounter with death at the concentration camp, an experience that affirmed his belief of the eternal soul, he became my first minister.

Because of this experience, he had collected hundreds of books on yoga and the religions of all cultures. Looking through his book collection, which had to be kept in large, padlocked trunks to protect them from my mother, became our favorite pastime. Reverently, we'd unlock the trunks and lift out the *Koran, The Aquarian Gospel of Jesus the Christ, The Secrets of the Egyptian Pyramids*. There were books on the Aztecs, the Greeks, and Raja Yoga; books on Confucianism, Buddhism, astral travel, and mind concentration.

"They are all saying the same thing," my father instructed me. "They are all searching for God, which isn't anywhere outside. It's within." Reading my father's books, I saw that Jesus, the Buddha, the rabbis, and the native shamans of aboriginal cultures all used stories as a primary tool for teaching people about moral conduct and spiritual peace. Stories allow the listener to be an active participant in his education by discovering the meaning of the lesson for himself.

When my older sister Nancy turned 19, my mother threw her out of the house, and she became a Hare Krishna devotee. As Narada-Dasi, Nancy preached the ideas of Krishna non-stop. For many years, her transformation embarrassed me, and I didn't listen, but later I tackled Hindu mythology on my own and studied Krishna, Vishnu, Radha, Ganesha, Kali, and other gods and goddesses.

The inspirational and philosophical qualities of all these "stories" got me through my difficult childhood. They gave me hope and an anchor for my foundering life. I still struggled through my teens and early twenties, but over time and with practice, I learned to use *svadyaya*, or self-study, to understand the source of my anger and deeply engrained negative self-talk. I saw how I suffered from my mother's fears and her own self-hatred, and I learned to find compassion for her. I forgave her. With practice, I recognized when I was not telling the truth about myself and how this caused me to suffer. I realized how much I hurt myself with negative self-talk, self-hatred, and lack of self-confidence.

In my study, I discovered that a story was a guide. Its symbols pointed to that eternal truth within that cannot be understood by the mind but only experienced in the heart. Over time, with physical asana, meditation, and storytelling, I realized how much my slant on life relied on my mind's somewhat random interpretation of my experiences. By identifying with this *ahamkara*, or ego, I was covering up my true nature, the *atman*. When I practiced such a path to self-knowledge as yoga, I could return to my eternal and ever present self.

Most of all, I realized that the story I created from my life and carried around all these years was just that, only a story. All I had was the eternal present, and from here I could create anything.

Years later, my yoga and meditation training helped me brave another difficult time. After his business went bankrupt, my first husband committed suicide. There was not a penny in the bank account. I had to sell all of our cars and most of my possessions; the house went into foreclosure. Homeless and jobless, I found myself the single caretaker of my five-year-old son and two-year-old daughter.

Although I felt traumatized, my yoga and meditation practice had prepared me to deal with the upheaval by embracing the present moment and carefully watching my mind's fears. During this period of grief, I started Storytime Yoga with the mission to educate children in yoga through story by offering them tools for mental and physical health.

While I was writing this book, my nine-year-old son, Alejandro, continued to grieve over the suicide of his father. He wanted to know why his Dad killed himself — how he could do such a thing. One night, I finally told him that his father committed suicide because his business went bankrupt and that it's hard for men in our culture to fail, especially financially. I explained, however, that not all people kill themselves over failure. I said that Daddy was very sad inside and very sick to do something like that.

Then I told him my story about growing up. Previously, I had shared the funny, happy stories of my youth, but now I thought it wise to tell him the darker stories. I wanted him to know that difficult things happen to all people: someone dies, someone is violent — but we can be strong, courageous, loving, peaceful and kind in the face of any difficulty. With our stories and our yoga, we can understand the fears, hurts, and desires that keep us hidden from our true selves, which is perfect and eternal.

Alejandro, along with his sister Paloma, had always come to the yoga classes I taught, but when he was eight, he chose to stop taking classes. Although he was still participating in our family practice of Storytime Yoga™ and meditation, he needed a break from the pressures of performing as the teacher's child. But after I shared these two difficult passages with him — my emergence from a dysfunctional home and his father's suicide — and reminded him of the calm and peace that comes from looking at the mind in meditation, Alejandro chose to rejoin the class of eight- to twelve-year-olds.

As for my student Brian — one year after he began coming to my after-school yoga class, he demonstrated a new confidence in his ability to find peace in an unbalanced environment. He told me that while his parents watched television, he did sun salutations. Proudly, he showed me his strong locust pose. During meditation, he was both eager and focused. He cited heroes from our stories, such as the little boy in *Children of Wax* and the nun in *Cherry Blossoms*, who made him feel good about himself and gave him the courage to face his world.

In our fast-paced society, we are often alienated from each other and our true selves, and we suffer needlessly. In pursuit of rationality, our minds have locked the doors to our hearts. But, like Brian, when we look inward with the disciplines of yoga and story, we can begin to distinguish the causes of our suffering and weed them out of the garden of the heart.

May there be peace in your heart, and may there be peace on earth.

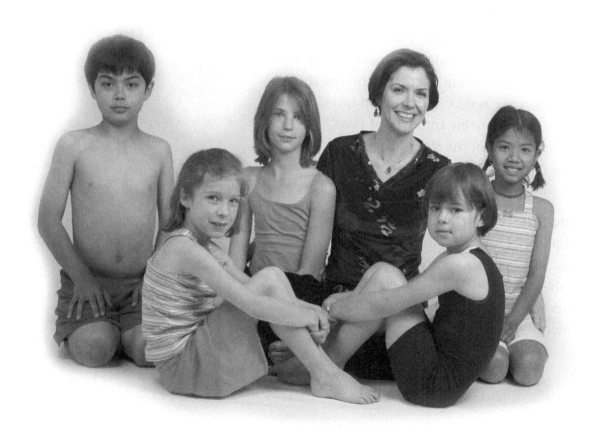

How to Use This Book

You can use Storytime Yoga™ stories in the classroom or at home. It is recommend for use with children between ages 8 and 12, however, you can adapt it for younger children by reading the instructions in the Joy of Stories chapter. Here are few ideas to get you started.

WITH YOGA ASANA

Tell the story as part of a yoga class and act it out with yoga poses (asanas). This method is outlined in my first book, *Storytime Yoga™: Teaching Yoga to Children Through Story*. It contains ideas for a complete yoga class, many techniques for teaching yoga with story, and photographs of yoga poses. For more yoga poses, consult BKS Iyengar's classic *Light on Yoga*. Also, try *Yoga Journal* and *Yoga + Joyful Living* magazines.

AS A THEME

Tell the story at the beginning of class and use it as a theme throughout the class. For instance, the story *Standing Still* is about finding stillness within. Allow children to contemplate this story and the theme as they do yoga asanas. Continue to bring up the story and its theme throughout class. Bring the essence of the story into the practice of each pose.

DURING RELAXATION

Tell the story at the beginning or end of class with relaxation or yoga nidra. I call these "story siestas," and children tend to have excellent retention with this method.

BY ITSELF

Tell the story by itself. For instructional purposes, I have applied meaning to each story. It's not necessarily what the listener may think the story is about, but only my interpretation. The listener's may be completely different. You can ask children what they think the story means. Using the method "Think, Pair, Share," have children think about their answer, pair up to discuss their observations, and then share them with the class. Have children write, draw pictures, or do other expressive work with the stories and share their creations. Additionally, you can tell the stories at bedtime, dinnertime, in the car, waiting in line at the grocery store, or as a special time.

IN YOUR OWN AUDIOS

You can create your own audios by recording the stories with your voice. Have children read along with the story after hearing it once.

WITH PERSONAL STORIES

Be sure to tell children personal stories about your experiences that relate to the stories. Children love to hear stories of their family, and it creates a powerful bond. When you share authentically about yourself, you move them to a deeper reflection about themselves. Ultimately, they will be inspired to tell their own stories.

More Ideas

- Have children relax and listen to the story first without the words or pictures.

- Ask children to draw a picture of some of the images and events from the story that they "saw" with their imaginations.

- Have children retell the story or the part of the story they illustrated. They can write it down if they wish. Younger children can dictate as you write their words down.

- Encourage children to tell the story to friends and family.

- Ask children to compare and contrast their retelling with that of the written story.

- Have children make a list of the images and characters in the story. Ask them to relate each image or character to their own lives. For example, in the story the *Roar of Awakening*, ask them how they are like the young tiger cub, the motherly goat, and the old wise tiger. Ask them what qualities these characters have that are like their own personality. Ask them if they know other people with or without these qualities.

- Have children relate the action or problem to their life story. Ask them if they have had a similar experience in life. Ask them how they can make changes or improve their lives.

- Have children make up their own story with the theme or characters from the story, and add yoga poses to it.

- Yoga Theater: Have children act out the stories as a theatrical play, complete with yoga asanas.

- Have children draw a symbol of what one story means to them. Have them share that meaning with the class.

- Have children draw, paint, sculpt or write a poem to express what a story means to them.

- Ask children to contemplate the story throughout their day. Does the story's meaning change for them? Does life ever mirror the story? What else arises? Ask them to be aware of this inner space where things arise as they carry the story with them.

- Ask children to keep track of their dreams at night after contemplating the story or yoga practice. Have them tell their dreams, draw pictures of the symbols, and contemplate the symbols.

- Have children keep a personal yoga journal to keep track of feelings, dreams, wishes, stories, and asanas.

The Joy of Stories

Want to hold a four-year-old's attention? Tell him a story! How about a restless 8-year-old? Tell her a story! Children love stories, and the more you tell them, the more they will ask for them. By creating their own images from the stories they hear, children develop the imagination and self-awareness. A child needs to have an inner life rich with symbols and a connection to the depth of the unconscious before he can climb the stairs into the intellect. With these tools, he can retrieve the treasures of the unconscious within to help him deal with the rational world of the mind and the material world around him. Listening to stories leads to critical thinking, self-reliance, and originality, all of which are essential for learning. By telling the story orally, rather than reading it, you will create an intense connection to your children.

Storytelling is very simple. It is not essential that you memorize any text. Instead, familiarize yourself with a series of images that you will use to retell the story. Remember: it's okay to make up your own version. To tell a story, memorize the beginning line. Then thread images together. What happens next? What is the next image that comes to your mind? Connect these images like pearls on a necklace. Memorize the ending sentence. Have the story come alive with words that use colors, sounds, scents, and other details. Speak loudly and with lots of expression. Exaggerate your facial expressions and vary the pitch, tone and rhythm of your voice to make the story interesting. Move your body!

"it is essential to engage the audience with interaction"

When telling a story to preschoolers, it is essential to engage the audience with interaction. Engage children in clapping hands, snapping fingers, pounding feet, wiggling, roaring like tigers. For this age group, choose a simple story and tell it in simple terms. Focus on the characters and their essential actions without too much detail.

I also encourage interaction with older children. Ask them questions: "So what do you think? Should the peddler go on his journey? Why or why not?" For older kids, you should take the time to paint the story with your words and images. Create special voices for each character, make up a special movement or sound each time a character enters, and encourage children to participate by performing the movement or sound to help you with the story.

You can take any story and pull out the bare bones of it. Who is the story about? What happens? What happens next? How does it end? Look for the three Rs – Rhyme, Rhythm, and Repetition. Make up a funny repetitive sound that goes with the story. It can be as simple as calling out "OH, YEAH!" every time a character appears, or you might try a more complex call and response.

Children love chants. Here's one from the story The Roar of Awakening:

> LITTLE GOAT, LITTLE GOAT
> NOPE, NOPE, NOPE, NOPE
> I AM A TIGER BIG AND STRONG
> I AM A TIGER ALL ALONG

I like to use props with my storytelling. I keep them in a special story bag and pull them out in front of the class one at a time. Children know Lalita the Marequita, a ladybug puppet who speaks Spanish and recites nonsense poetry; Marequita sets the rules for our group interaction. Then there is Mr. Bones, a rubber skeleton that emphasizes healthy eating and teaches anatomy. Sophia, the Snake of Dreams, asks children about the dreams they had last night. I also have glockenspiels and bells, which draw children's attentions in like magic. Those who are good at controlling their bodies and listening get the reward of ringing the bells!

I always act stories out dramatically with any age group. I am the silliest with preschoolers, and it's so much fun! I make exaggerated facial expressions and strange sounding noises for characters. I use my whole body, and children focus on it. I've done classes with 50 preschoolers, and teachers come up to me and say, "How did you get them to be so still?" I tell them it was all in the power of story, imagery, and their own imaginations, spellbinding them into finding the world within their own bodies. The same thing happens with older kids. Connect to them with story, and you will have their attentions and hearts.

Techniques for Teaching Yoga Philosophy to Children

For preschool children, simply teaching kindness, non-harming, and courage is teaching yoga philosophy. Kindergartners are becoming self-aware and can begin to relate the shorter stories to their own lives; eight- to twelve-years-olds can grasp longer stories and the concepts behind them. With the younger age group, I discuss the concept of non-attachment, and to the older children, I introduce the word *aparigraha*, which means non-attachment.

The following are techniques that I use for children five years and older to help them see themselves beyond their story of who they are. I frequently use one of these techniques at the beginning of the class, reinforce the idea in the story I tell, and refer back to it during our practice of the asanas.

1) CREATING INTENTIONS

At the start of class, I talk about intentions. Intentions are better than goals because intentions can change with time, and unlike goals, they carry no frustrating expectations of achievement. Setting an intention helps focus the mind and move toward the desired result, while allowing for flexibility according to what's happening in the present moment. An intention can be to have fun, to be calm, to be more flexible.

Have children write down their intention. Then have them say it out loud to the class. By saying the intention, they are actually creating it. The word God comes from the Proto-Indo-European word *ghut*, which means "to call forth, to invoke." The word invoke means to use the voice. So when we are using our voices, we are creating like God.

2) USING PUPPETS

I love puppets, and so do children of every age. To introduce the title and theme of the story, I use a pirate puppet given to me by an old friend. The pirate helps the children identify the background of the story: the country, religion, or perhaps culture and theme of the story. You can find a great selection of puppets at www.Folkmanis.com.

3) YOK-A – CONNECTING TO YOU!

I teach that yoga means union, and that it comes from the Sanskrit word *"yug,"* or to yoke. Our English word for yoke comes from this word, like the yoke on an ox. Tell children that we are doing YOK-A, or yoking to our true selves and our talents and gifts and bringing them to the world. Regardless of religious beliefs, children can "yoke" or find a central still point within themselves that they can rest in, as well as "yoke" to any preferred deity, or not.

4) THE SUN AND THE CLOUD

Our true nature, our inner self or being is like the sun, I tell the children. It is singular, brilliant, everlasting, and central. But our minds are like a cloud, which sometimes covers the sun and blocks it. We forget that there is a sun behind the cloud and focus only on the cloud. The discipline of yoga can help us move the cloud out of the way, so that we can again identify with the radiant self and all its possibilities. When we separate with the mind and its "story," we blow the cloud out of the way. Have the children watch their thinking and act out the blowing to remove the cloud from their minds.

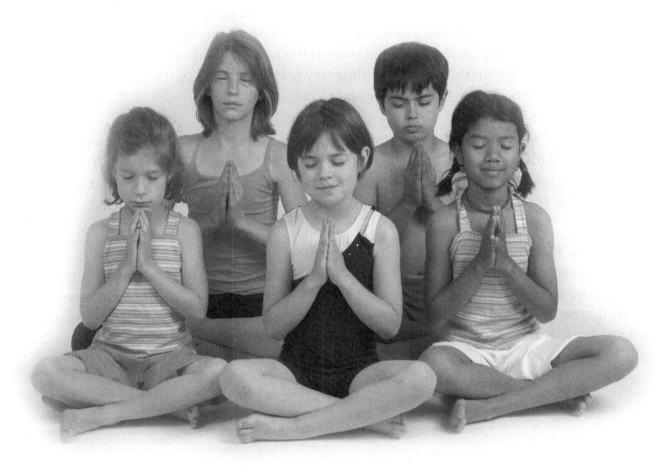

5) THE ONION

The psychologist Carl Jung compared the self to an onion. At the core of the onion is our true self. However, things happen to us in life, and our minds make meaning and story out of it. Each meaning we place on ourselves is like a layer of the onion, little by little, covering up our true nature. Instead of identifying with our true selves, we identify with boy or girl, black or white, rich or poor, lucky or unlucky. This identification with the ego self — the layers of the onion — is what hides us from our true self. With the discipline of yoga, we can begin to peel back the layers. Acting out the peeling away of the layers of an imaginary onion is helpful. Make a fist and peel away each finger saying, "not me, not me." Then say, "but then" and open the fist and reveal the emptiness in your hand without saying anything more. With the smallest children, you can reveal a small jewel.

6) THE TRAINED PUPPY

The mind is like an untrained puppy. There may be a big pork chop awaiting the puppy down a path, but the puppy is sniffing and looking at everything on the edges of the path, looking here and looking there, making a zigzag in his progress. It will take the puppy a long time to find his goal. With time and training, the puppy will become disciplined and go straight to the pork chop without being distracted by all the scents around him. Tell children that yoga can get you to your goal faster and make life easier. Have the children act out the sniffing puppy and the wiser, trained puppy.

7) WHAT I WANT MOST IN THE WHOLE WORLD

Ask children what they want most in the world. Someone will say all the food in the world, another child will want to fly, someone will want to live in California, and someone will want a horse. Tell them that all their dreams are possible with the discipline of yoga. Instead of being like the puppy dog, which is distracted by everything along the path, we can use yoga to help us stay focused on our dream.

8) SPACE IN BETWEEN THE THOUGHTS

Our minds are important to us. We don't want to stop thinking entirely; besides, it's impossible! But we need to rest our thoughts, so I use this exercise to teach children how to rest in the space between their thoughts. First, have children become aware of their breath, breathing in and out, in and out. When they think a thought, have them label that thought as "thinking," and then bring their awareness back to the breath. When I tell my students that we are trying to make space in between our thoughts, I exaggerate that sentence by making long pauses in between the words.
Space..........in............between...........our...........thoughts.

9) STAYING PRESENT

The present is all that we have. Something happened, or something is going to happen, but it's not happening now, so it doesn't exist. All that exists is now. To illustrate the present moment, I use the *namaste* position. I tell my students that the left hand is the past; the right hand is the future. When we bring our hands together into *namaste*, we rest the mind and breath in the space between the two hands, and this space is the present moment.

We can think of the past and the future as stories, but thinking about these stories requires energy, energy that takes us away from the powerful present. I explain to my students that energy is like a bank account; whenever we waste our energy on past or future thoughts (or any negative thought), we are spending money out of our account. To increase our bank accounts, we need to focus in the present and stay positive.

10) MONKEY STEALING THE JEWEL

Once children have learned the importance of staying in the present moment, I use the illustration of the monkey and the jewel to show them how to bring back a wandering mind. When my mind wanders, it's as if a silly little monkey has come and swiped the precious jewel of my present moment, the moment that gives me wisdom and power. With the namaste position, I bring back my awareness and take the jewel back from the monkey. Bring the monkey right back to the space where the two hands meet— the present.

11) THE HEROIC JOURNEY

I tell my students that we are on a hero's journey, and that journey leads into ourselves. On this journey, treading the path of yoga, we will find the great treasure within us and bring it out as our gift to the world. Like other heroes, we will face demons on our sojourn: bad habits, impatience, and desires. Yoga is the tool we use to fight our demons, and like the heroes in our stories, we must do many battles. But with the heart-felt courage we learn from the old woman in *The Jewel in the Well* and with the determination and patience of the river in *The Story of the Sands*, we will prevail.

> *"we are on a hero's journey, and that journey leads into ourselves"*

12) AWAKE IN THE WORLD

Teach children how to "stop" during their day. Have them become completely aware of the present moment and the witness consciousness that they possess. They might repeat, "I know that I am aware. I know that I am walking, brushing my teeth, getting dressed." As they become aware of time passing and things changing, they should realize that they are still present, aware and watching.

13) WALKING MEDITATION

In this meditation, students form a line and join the ends into a circle, so that each student faces the back of the student in front of him. They wrap their right hands around their left fists and walk very slowly as they notice their breathing, in and out. This is a slow, careful walk: stepping heel-to-toe with the front foot, then pressing off with the ball of the back foot. Tell the children to focus on their feet in the earth, their hands around their fists. They should notice the passing of each step. As they walk, they might repeat silently to themselves, *I know that I am walking; I know that I am breathing in and breathing out.* This exercise increases a child's awareness that he is always here, although time passes and the forms occupying space change. Underlying everything, there is the self.

14) WHO AM I?

Encourage the children to question themselves: *Who am I? Who is the watcher of the thoughts I am thinking?* As they contemplate this over time, students will discover that they are not their minds, but something greater and everlasting.

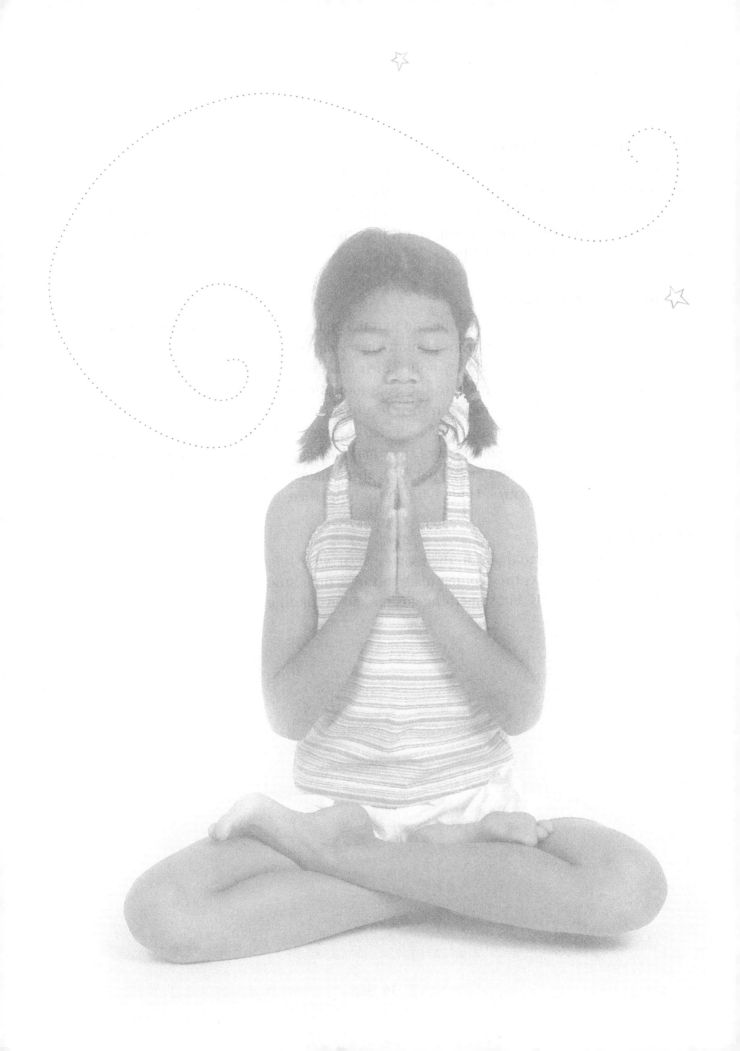

Relaxation for Children Through Yoga Nidra and Story

More and more, I hear children say that their biggest challenge is "needing to relax." With the busy schedule many kids keep — going to school; participating in sports and other extracurricular activities; keeping up with homework, chores, and church; and family activities — there is little time to unwind. The little down time available is often punctuated with the distractions of television, video games, and loud music.

Each yoga class should include some sort of *shavasana*, or relaxation. With every age group, I use a variant of Yoga Nidra, or sleep yoga, which helps children relax by using imagery and body awareness.

Paramhansa Swami Satyananda Saraswati, the founder of the Bihar School of Yoga in India, developed Yoga Nidra. Called sleep yoga, Yoga Nidra brings the mind into a deep state that is beyond dreaming, sleeping, and waking states. In Saraswati's book, *Yoga Nidra*, there are numerous studies that show Yoga Nidra's effectiveness for various illnesses, such as ADHD, cancer, and depression.

Yoga Nidra uses a rotation of consciousness, allowing the mind to rest on different body parts successively. Afterwards, a series of rapid images is given, and the *sankalpa*, or resolve, is used. One child's resolve might be "I am calm." Another person might affirm "I am loved." Like affirmations, *sankalpas* are used in the present tense.

I learned Yoga Nidra at Naropa University with my teacher Sreedevi Bringi, who studied at the Bihar School of Yoga. From her teachings, Saraswati's book, and my experience in teaching hundreds of children, I have adapted Yoga Nidra for children for classroom use.

The form for adults takes about 30 minutes. For children ages three to twelve, I adjust this time period accordingly. Most preschool children, as well as many older children, will wiggle around. This is fine; they are being exposed to relaxation and just beginning to create their own practice. However, if you want to reduce wiggling, you can offer a reward, such as ringing the bell, getting a sticker, or teaching a segment of the class.

Sometimes I use Yoga Nidra at the beginning of the class. I notice that in after-school programs, kids are tired after a long day at school, and often, they have just had a snack.

The relaxation and story let them unwind their busy minds, relax their bodies, and digest their food as they prepare for a yoga session.

I drop in a short story in the process of Yoga Nidra, allowing the children's imagination to arise within their bodies. I call this activity a "story siesta." The story siestas enhance creative learning, develop confidence and self-esteem, lower stress, improve focus and attention, and give relaxation to the body and mind.

SIMPLIFIED VERSION OF YOGA NIDRA FOR CHILDREN

- Find a quiet place with dimmed lights, but not total darkness. There should be no interruptions. Children lie on their backs with their arms slightly away from the body, palms facing up. To reduce distractions, I encourage them to cover their eyes with a beanie baby or a washcloth or even a sock.

- I use a small glockenspiel during relaxation, which helps children focus and relax. I play random notes to my liking, and children have told me how much they enjoy it, how much it helps them focus; some even have the feeling of leaving their body.

- Have children focus on their breathing. Begin with three deep breaths. Inhale saying "yes" to life; then exhale, letting go and dropping into the earth.

- Have children think of a simple *sankalpa*: For example, "I am healthy. I am calm."

- Have children tighten all body muscles, one at a time, and then relax them. Make a fist with the right hand, tense the right arm, hold; and let go. Do the same with the left hand and arm, the right foot and leg, the left foot and leg, the chest, the lower back, and the shoulders. Press the tongue against the roof of the mouth, scrunch up the face, hold, and let go. After they've tightened and relaxed each successive part of the body, tense the entire body, hold, and let go.

- Tell them to imagine the sun on a beautiful beach (you can substitute the moon or another image of light). Allow the light from that sun to touch each body part as it is called out. Imagine it filled with golden light. Beginning with the toes, proceed to name each body part, such as heel, ankle, entire foot, calf, knee, thigh, hips, stomach, chest, back, neck, shoulders, arms, elbows, hands, fingers, neck, chin, jaw, lips, cheeks, eyes, whole head, whole body. For older children you can get more detailed, such as front of knee, back of knee, front of arm, armpit.

FOR PRESCHOOL

- Allow two to five minutes for the Yoga Nidra session.

- Imagine the sun touching the parts of the body: feet, legs, hips, chest, arms, hands, neck, jaw, cheeks, lips, eyes, nose, and ears; the whole head; and the whole body. Relax.

- Call out images, such as a rose, a candle, a tall mountain.

- Make a suggestion such as "I am peaceful," "I am relaxed," "I feel safe."

- Return to silence.

- Return awareness to the outside world, let them stretch, rock, roll over to their right side and rest before using their arms to get up.

- Let children talk about their experiences and what they "saw and felt" within.

- Have them draw pictures and make up stories around the images. Transcribe their words onto paper.

FOR K-2

- Expand the Yoga Nidra session to five to ten minutes.

- Add more body parts, such as back of knee, armpit. Tell them to imagine the space between their lips, the space between their eyelids and eyes, the space between their body and the floor. Drop in imagery, such as a rose, a candle, a rushing river, and then tell a short story without the glockenspiel.

- Use a *sankalpa* such as "I love myself," "I am whole and complete," "My ideas matter."

- Return to silence.

- Ring a bell to bring the children's awareness back to the room. Let them stretch, rock, roll over to their right side and rest for a moment before using their arms to get up.

- Ask the children what they saw and felt. They might want to write about their experience or draw their feelings.

FOR CHILDREN EIGHT TO TWELVE YEARS OLD

- Take 10-15 minutes for the session, and use more body parts. At this age, I also work with the left and right sides of the body. For example, tell them to tense the right toes, right ankle, right foot, right calf, and so on, up the right side of the body; then the left toes, and so on. On the face, take more time with the left eye, right eye, right eyebrow, left eyebrow, and so on.

- Use a longer story or a fairy tale. The story and imagery, told in a soft tone, will keep them focused on the body through the imagination.

- Try a more detailed guided imagery. For instance, have them imagine a treasure chest at the heart level. Ask them to decorate that chest with their imagination; then open it a crack and see the golden light pouring out. Ask them to experience this light as it touches the toes, legs, arms. Open the lid of the chest wider and look inside. Ask them what is there? What gifts do they have? Give them examples, such as the gift of helping their mother, or the gift of art and math, or the gift of making people laugh. Tell them to smile at their treasures and make a wish for themselves, their family, their school, and the world.

- Return to silence.

- Ring a bell to bring awareness back to the room. Tell the children to stretch, rock, roll over to their right side, and rest before using their arms to get up.

- Ask the children what they saw and felt. Like the younger children, they may want to write or draw their experience. They can also create their own visualizations.

RECOMMENDED BOOKS FOR STORY SIESTAS

Satyananda recommends stories such as those from the *Puranas*. There are also wonderful stories from the *Panchatantra*, Aesop, and Jataka Tales.

ALL AGES *Peace Tales* by Margaret Read McDonald, *One Hand Clapping Zen Stories* for All Ages by Rafe Martin, *Stories to Nourish the Hearts of Our Children in a Time of Crisis* by Laura Simms, *The Children's Book of Virtues* by William J. Bennett, *The Soul's Almanac: A Year of Interfaith Stories, Prayers and Wisdom* by Aaron Zerah, *Doorways to the Soul* by Elisa Pearmain, *Wisdom Stories from Around the World* by Heather Forest. *Parabola* Magazine also has wonderful short stories: www.Parabola.org.

FOR OLDER CHILDREN *The Great Fairytale Tradition* by Jack Zipes, *Fearless Girls Wise Women and Beloved Sisters* by Kathleen Ragan, *Favorite Folktales from Around the World* by Jane Yolen. Any Grimm's fairytale book.

Creating Your Own Guided Visualizations for Children

Bringing imagination to a child's world is one of the most important things we can do. The Greeks said that the soul speaks in images. It is the *imago dei*, or image of God, that arises from the heart and connects us to the divine within.

I always teach yoga with a theme of story, which is either acted out with the yoga postures or brought up as a theme throughout the class. Before relaxation, allow children to call out the images that came to them during the story — those "pictures in my head." They can draw a symbol for an image, and tell about what it means to them or how it relates to the story.

Use a variant of Yoga Nidra for children to get them to relax. Begin with awareness of the sounds in the room and awareness of their breathing. Then call out certain body parts, such as the feet, the knees. This rotation of consciousness allows the busy mind to rest on the body and eventually relax into a deeper state. For the youngest children in pre-school, make this very short — feet, legs, hips, chest. For older children, you can take more time in calling out body parts — toes, ankle, foot, and so on.

Then guide the children to drop their awareness down to their heart center. Here you can either drop in a symbol from the story or allow the children to use the symbol they created from the story. Or, you can drop in any image you create — a ship sailing on the seas, a rose blooming, a bird in flight, a river rushing through a canyon. Allow children to create images that are appealing to them. What do they like? What makes them happy? Allow them to imagine people they love.

With their imaginations, you can also have them revisit the story you told as if they were the main character of the story. Have the child visualize the story again as the character. Ask them questions during the visualization, such as what do you see? Where are you? You can pull out main elements of the story and ask them to connect them to their lives: What journey are you on? What do you want in your life? What obstacle do you have in your life? What animal friend do you have in your life? What can you do to get help? Allow the child to let things arise, without forcing anything. Teach them to rest their minds in the space between the thoughts to allow things to arise between the thoughts.

You can create guided visualizations by starting one off on a journey — starting with a place, such as a forest, outer space, a boat sailing to an island. Have them imagine the place in detail. What sounds, smells, and sights do they see? You can add characters, such as an animal guide, a fairy, a person who greets them. What happens next? Have them reach a special place. What is it? A bubbling pot, a magic door, a secret well? What comes out of it? What message is there for them? What image, object, animal is just for them? Have them return, saying goodbye and returning with a magical object that was found. Try to provide them with a feeling of safety, comfort, joy, or relaxation.

Allow the child to "talk" to the characters in their visualization. What do they say? Encourage children to do this exercise after relaxation as well, by writing down the conversation. This is called active imagination and can help children learn to problem solve. Adults can do this too!

Design the visualization to solve a problem. If there is some anxiety, let children jump off a cliff in their mind's eye to learn to let go. Let them feel the falling freely and safely. Let them enter a cave of darkness safely and find magical gifts. What are the gifts? What magical abilities to they have to solve the problem they are having? If they need to relax, allow them to just sink into the earth. Perhaps they will journey into another world. Allow them to drop into this and play with whatever arises for them.

Have them invite a symbol to come from within to help them remember how to let go, to be courageous, to be relaxed. Encourage them to remember that symbol, let it rest in their heart, and know that it is available at any time they need it. Have them draw the personal symbol, and suggest that they put it in a place where they can see it every day.

You can guide them with an intention, such as expansion, connectedness, love for others, or gratitude. Ask them to think about images of expansion, love, and gratitude that are in their own lives. For example, with expansion, you could create a visualization that awareness expands from their heart, out to their toes, out to the floor, to the person next to them, to the door, out the door. You could use the same visualization for connectedness.

Another way to enter into guided visualization is to find an opening or door in the mind's eye. Perhaps it is an oak tree, and there is a door there. Perhaps it is a hole in the earth, or a looking glass. Where do you go? Down or up? What happens? What feelings arise as you enter?

Upon entering such a place, children can influence their surroundings. If they need healing in any part of their body, have them imagine little workers, or any other image for them, repairing their body. If there is something they desire, have them visualize them doing the desired action, or having the desired object.

During meditation, ask children to create an affirmation in the positive, such as, I am smart, I am kind. I am confident. Have them repeat it three times to themselves during meditation. Have them visualize an image to represent this affirmation.

Allow children to choose a Spirit Animal — Some special animal that they may have dreamed about or see a lot in waking life with which they have a special affinity. Let the Spirit Animal guide them somewhere. Where is it? What does the Spirit Animal say? Let the child become the animal. If it is a raven, ask the child to fly and see where it goes.

In my book *Storytime Yoga™: Teaching Yoga to Children Through Story*, I have fairy tale *shavasana* for older children. Each successive relaxation allows a child to journey on an original fairy tale.

- Who is in the story? What happens in the character's life that they are called on a journey? What has been upset in the character's life that must be brought back into balance, healed, defeated?

- What is it that must be restored to bring life back into balance, healed, or vindicated?

- What secrets are there? What animals or magical helpers come their way?

- What obstacles must be overcome? What magical objects are discovered to overcome the obstacles?

- How is the problem overcome? What is the action that overcomes the problem?

- How does it end?

After the visualizations, encourage children to draw, write and speak about the images they saw. Encourage children to contemplate the images throughout their day. Have them pay attention to their dreams and keep a dream journal. Have them draw their dreams.

Encourage them to be aware of the images in their waking life, such as animals, flowers, keys and doors, certain people, and so on, to relate them symbolically to their own lives. This cultivates attention to the present and reflection on what's going on inside and how it relates to their life on the outside.

Encourage children to monitor their thoughts. To listen to that inner voice, the chatter. Remind children that they are not their thoughts. They are something much more than their thoughts.

Above all, encourage children to practice meditation and relaxation at home! Even to invite their parents and friends to join them!

As a teacher, in creating your own guided visualizations, your own imagination is the only limit! Teach out of your own experience. What are your issues and how can imagery and guided imagination help you? What would make you feel safe, help you cool down anger, or relax? What great adventures, joys do you have? Create your own visualizations and then use them on children. We are all human and have the same hopes and fears, joys and sorrows. You can connect deeper to your children when you share from your own experience and offer up to them the healing and joy you have received. Images are universal and it is the individual who will receive messages for his or her own life's needs. That is the connection of the outer to the inner, and the inner to the eternal.

The Treasure in Your Heart

The Stories

The stories in this series are labeled as treasures for inward exploration and development. These treasures can't be found in the material world; they can't be bought or stolen or lost. These treasures — courage, kindness, belief in the self, understanding the mind, controlling anger, sacrificing for others and more — come from within. When we find these gifts inside ourselves, we are able to share them with everyone around us and ultimately create a more peaceful world. I have scripted this section of the book so that an instructor or a participant may read the story and work directly with the related asanas and meditations.

TREASURE: Self-Reliance

THE JEWEL IN THE WELL - Unknown

There was once an old woman who went every day to a deep well to fetch some water. One day when she drew up her bucket, her eye caught something glimmering at the bottom of the bucket. She fished it out and found that it was a large, stunning ruby that flashed brightly in the sun's ray.

"My, my," she said. "Isn't that a beauty?" Without another thought, she dropped the jewel into her purse, then sat down to eat her lunch and drink her water.

A young man came by the well. He sat down beside the old woman with a terribly worried look on his face.

"Is there anything the matter, young man?" the old woman asked.

"Oh, yes, I have many problems," he said. "I can't find any work in my home town, so I must go far to another town for work to feed my family. Life is so difficult." He started to fetch some water from the well when the old woman had an idea. She reached into her purse and found the ruby.

"Here," she said to the man. "Take this. Perhaps it will help you on your journey."

The man was amazed. "You are giving this to me?"

"Yes, take it," she said. "You need it more than I do."

The young man was overwhelmed by her gift. He thanked her again and again before he set off for the next town.

A few weeks later, the old woman went to her well as usual, and the young man was there again.

"Hmmm, is there something else that you want?" the old woman said. "Didn't things work out in the new town?"

"Oh, yes, everything went very well, thanks to you and that jewel you gave me. But I want something else from you, he said. "I want it very badly."

"What is it?" she asked.

"I want that which you have within you that was able to give that precious jewel to me — a total stranger — without a thought. That is what I truly need."

WORKING WITH THE STORY

ACTIVITIES

Contemplate this story during asana practice, meditation, or relaxation.

What does the old woman have? Where does she find it? How did she get it?

Have you ever given away something you really liked? How did it feel? What kinds of things do you do to help others?

What do you think about money? Where does it come from? Do you have enough? How do you know how much is enough?

What does it mean to trust? How can we trust that whatever we need in life will be supplied? What is the difference between a want and a need?

ASANA

To work with uncertainty try these constricted poses. Although we may not know what's going on behind us, for life turns us upside down, we can take comfort in the breath as time passes in the pose. We can trust within that all things will work out.

PLOW POSE — *Halasana*
SEATED FORWARD BEND — *Pashimotanasana*
HEADSTAND — *Salamba Sirsasana*

SHAVASANA AND MEDITATION

Visualize a deep well. See the well and its deep blackness. Don't be afraid of that blackness or its emptiness. Reach into the well. What is there? Is it a jewel? A person? An animal? Some other object? What is its purpose? What does it say to you? What is it for?

TREASURE: The True Self

In this busy, materialistic world, we tend to forget who we are. We are conditioned, like the goat, to wander in a world of concepts and limitations. Like the goat, we follow the herd. Advertising tells us what to wear, what to buy, what to do, and what is important. We are trapped in ignorance of our true selves. Our true Self is not the goat; it is the tiger. It is the divine, unlimited, everlasting Self which resides in all beings, and all beings are One.

THE ROAR OF AWAKENING - Hindu

There was once a pregnant tigress that was ready to deliver her cub, but she was very hungry. She had been hunting for many days without success when she finally came upon a herd of grazing goats. So ravenous was her hunger that even though she was exhausted, she sprang into the herd of goats. This great leap prompted the birth throes, and from sheer exhaustion, she died on the spot.

But the tiger cub that was within her was born alive and well.

The little goats, being friendly and compassionate, gathered around him.

"Gaa, what have we here?" a mother goat said.

"I don't know, but let's take care of it!" said another. "Poor little thing!"

So the goats adopted the orphaned tiger cub as their own, nursed it along with their own offspring, and fondly watched over it.

By following the example of the little baby goats, the tiger cub learned how to eat grass. At first it was difficult for him to handle the thin blades of grass with his sharp teeth, but he figured it out. The vegetarian diet kept him slim, and his temperament became meek. Playing among the goats, he learned goat language. Eventually, he could let out a "blaaarraaa" bleat as well as anyone else. So of course he thought he was a goat.

One night, a fierce old male tiger approached the herd. The goats all scattered with fear. But the tiger cub, devoid of fear, remained where he was.

A young tiger among the goats? The old male tiger could not believe his eyes.

"What is this? A grass-eating tiger cub among goats! Ridiculous!"

"Graaaaaa" the tiger/goat cub bleated, and then plucked a piece of thin grass and chewed it.

"What is this nonsense?" The old tiger roared, enraged. "What are you doing among these silly goats? Why on earth are you eating grass?"

"Graaa," was all the tiger cub could say.

Furious, the old tiger grabbed him by the scruff of the neck and shook him, as if to knock him back to his senses. He carried the frightened cub down to a pool of water and sat him down next to it, forcing him to look into its mirrored surface, which was illuminated by the full moon.

"Look! Look, I say! Look into that pool of water and see our two faces. We are alike, you and I! You have the face of a fierce tiger, like mine. You are not a goat! You are a tiger, so why do you bleat like a goat and eat like a goat when you are not a goat? You are a tiger!"

The little cub stared at the images for a long time. He began to feel uneasy. Shifting from paw to paw, he let out another little "Graaaaa."

"Oh, for goodness sakes!" the old tiger exclaimed and carried the cub off to his den. There he gave the cub a piece of raw meat left over from an earlier meal.

But the cub shuddered with disgust.

"Here, take it and eat it!" the tiger commanded. "Chew it! Swallow it!" The cub began to chew and was just about to make another noise, when the taste settled on his tongue... hmmm. He began to feel an unfamiliar satisfaction as this new food went down to his belly. He felt a strange, glowing strength spreading throughout his whole body; he felt wonderful. He arose and gave a mighty yawn, as if he were waking from a long night's sleep. He stretched his body out; he arched his back; he extended his forelegs and spread his claws. Suddenly, his tail lashed the ground and from his throat burst the terrifying, triumphant ROAR of a tiger.

"Now do you know what you really are?" asked the old tiger. The young cub nodded, and then the two went out into the jungle to hunt together.

WORKING WITH THE STORY

ACTIVITIES

Contemplate this story during asana practice, meditation, or relaxation.

How are you like the tiger cub? Can you remember an experience where you didn't realize you had the strength or ability to do something? What is something that you'd like to achieve? How are you like the goat? Do you know any people who are like the goats? How are you like the old tiger? What qualities do the tigers and goats have that we can incorporate in our life?

Here is an exercise to help you become aware of the eternal Self within. At the beginning of class note, "Class is now beginning." Recall the things you did before class began perhaps you brushed your teeth, got ready for school, studied, or played with friends.

As time passes, forms arise and disappear. Our witness of the events, our true self, is always present and aware.

Soon, class will be over. We will go home, remember the day and the yoga class; however, we will still be "here." Notice at the end of the class that this was true; time did pass but we are still "here."

ASANA

Be the mother tiger with **WARRIOR I**, *virabhadrasana* I. Feel your strength. As the cub you become **DOWNWARD DOG**, *adho mukha svanasana*. The little goats are **UNICORN POSE**, *vashistasana*. Along comes the old tiger and you take **WARRIOR II**, *virabhadrasana II*. When the tiger take you to his cave, move to **UPWARD FACING BOW**, *urdva dhanurasana*. When you realize who you are, roar like a tiger! **LION POSE**, *simhasana*.

Notice the breath and the awareness that stays with us as we move to another pose.

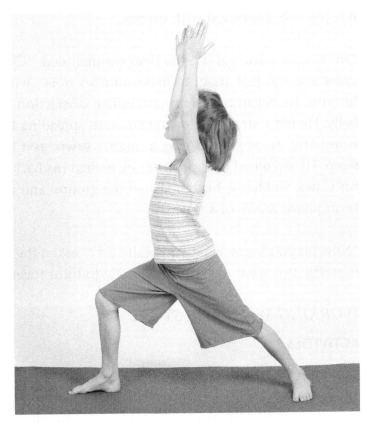

CHANT

> My heart is big and strong!
> I know that a great power resides in my heart!
> It is loving, fearless, kind and generous.

MEDITATION AND RELAXATION

Imagine a goat. As you picture the goat, think of all the things you cannot do, the things you haven't been able to achieve. What bothers you? What frustrates you? What is your, "I can't..."

Now visualize the tiger. Change the "I can't" phrase into "I can." Silently repeat to yourself the things you want to achieve, in the positive form, as "I can." Then repeat silently to yourself, "I am love; I am peace; I am. I am."

TREASURE: Unity

There is an underlying unity of all things; all things are connected. When we feel connected to the Self within and to others, we become fearless and peaceful. All fear comes from the ego, which believes that it is separate. This happens because we think of the "I, Me, and Mine." When we are relaxed in our centers and calm in our minds, we can feel our true selves in connection to the universe.

Our sense of separateness comes from the way we sense the world around us. Our thoughts and the stories we tell ourselves make us believe that we are separate. This belief is like fingers holding onto a curtain. We see the fingers in front of a curtain as separate because we do not see the attached hand behind the curtain. The same concept applies to people. We know that we have different shapes, races, sexes, religions, political views, but we are one human race.

This story helps us realize the unity of all things.

BRAHMA'S TEARS – Hindu

Hanuman was the Monkey King who rescued Sita from the demon Ravana. One day, Hanuman went to see Lord Brahma, the creator of the universe. But Lord Brahma was crying.

"My Lord, why are you crying? What is wrong?" Hanuman asked.

"Oh, my dear Hanuman," Brahma said. "I held the jewel of wisdom in my hands. It was so beautiful — how it glimmered in the sunlight. But alas, I dropped it, and the jewel shattered into millions of tiny pieces."

"I see, said Hanuman. "You dropped the jewel and it broke. Is that why you are crying?"

"No," Brahma replied. "I cry because everyone who found a piece of the jewel of wisdom believes that he has the only piece."

WORKING WITH THE STORY

ACTIVITIES

Contemplate this story during asana practice, meditation, or relaxation.

What do you think this story is about? Is there more than one way to be right? What is self-righteousness? What happens when we make others wrong? How do we feel if we are made wrong? We may be getting power and self-justification out of our need to be right, but we lose an important connection – our unity with others.

Make a list of ways people are different: skin color, hairstyle, language, clothing, manners. Then make a list of ways that people are the same: everyone laughs and cries, needs food and shelter. How does our society make people separate? How can we transform this separation and work toward unity?

Think of the moon. The moon appears to have its own light and change into phases — but not really! The moon's light is only an illusion created by the sun's light. Only the moon's relationship to the earth and sun creates what we call the phases of the moon; the moon is always just itself. Even though there are phases, there is still only one, unified cycle of the moon.

ASANA

When doing these yoga poses, notice how all the parts of the body work together. For example, in **TRIANGLE POSE**, *trikonasana*, observe the setting of the foundation with the feet and legs. The chest twists and opens, and then the arm and hand rise up, and then the head looks at the hand. Many movements make one pose. Notice the muscles working, the bones moving. Observe how the body functions as a whole, and then observe how the class functions as a whole.

You are a jewel. With an open heart, you are aligned with the universe. Try heart-opening poses, such as, **CAMEL**, *ustrasana*, and **BOW POSE**, *dhanurasana*. What other jewels can you make with your body using asana? What kind are they?

MEDITATION AND RELAXATION

Imagine a beautiful jewel inside the heart. This jewel of wisdom is within you. Using an in breath, let the jewel rise up from the heart to the brow chakra. Breathing out, let the entire body feel this wisdom. Return to the heart chakra and imagine that this jewel is shining brightly for all to see. People are touched by the light's rays of love, compassion, calm, and wisdom.

TREASURE: Non-Violence

The violence that we see outside in our world is a reflection of the violence that goes on inside of us. When we hurt one another, it's usually because we are feeling that same emotion toward ourselves. When we are peaceful inside, nothing disturbs us. If something upsets us, we have to look deeper to find out why we are upset. Perhaps it is because of some old wound or fear. We can examine this fear, name it, and let it go. That way it cannot cause another upset.

We want to treat others and ourselves with loving kindness, but that does not mean that we don't protect others and ourselves. There is a story from the Vedas about a monk who made a yearly visit to villages to teach. One day, as he was entering a village, he saw a large, menacing snake that was terrorizing the citizens. The monk had a chat with the snake and taught him to be kind to others. The following year when the monk made his visit to the village, he saw the same snake again, but it was almost unrecognizable. This once enormous, fierce, and frightening creature was skinny and bruised. The monk asked the snake what had happened.

"I have stopped terrorizing the village in order to not harm anyone," the snake said. "But now, children are taunting and hurting me. They throw rocks at me. I'm afraid to leave my hiding place to hunt for fear of them."

"I told you not to harm anyone," said the monk, "but I never told you not to hiss."

THE CRACKED POT – Hindu

Once there was a farmer, and every day he carried two pots down to the river to fetch water. Each pot hung on the end of a pole, which the farmer carried across his neck and shoulders. The first pot he carried on his right side. This pot was new and shiny and perfect in every way. The second pot he carried on his left side. Now this pot was older, so much older that it had a crack in its side.

Every day, the new pot brought back all the water the farmer had poured into it. But the cracked pot leaked out water in a little trail behind the farmer in his long walk back from the stream to his house. This went on day after day. The perfect pot brought all the water and was proud of its accomplishments. But the cracked pot kept only about half of its water.

The little cracked pot began to feel terrible about itself. "There's something wrong with me," the cracked pot thought. "The perfect pot brings back all the water. My master gets all his effort's worth. However, I am only capable of bringing half his effort. I am so ashamed of my imperfection!"

After two years, the little cracked pot could stand it no longer.

Feeling like a failure, he spoke to the farmer. "Master, I am so ashamed. I must apologize to you. I have only been able to deliver half my load because this crack in my side leaks out water all the way back to your house. My terrible flaw causes you to get only half the value of your work. You should just get rid of me!"

The farmer said to the pot, "Little pot, do not despair. Look behind you. Do you not see those beautiful flowers along the path I walk every day? They are on the left side, where I carry you. They are not on my right side. Little pot, I have always known about your special feature. So I planted flower seeds along the path to the stream, and you have watered those seeds as I walked home. Thanks to you, every day for two years I have had fresh flowers for my table. Thank you, little cracked pot. You are very special."

WORKING WITH THE STORY

ACTIVITIES

Contemplate this story during asana practice, meditation, or relaxation.

Do you sometimes have negative thoughts about your abilities? How does that feel? Can you substitute positive thoughts for the negative ones? How do you do this?

Observe yourself during asana practice. Are you forcing a pose? Are you judging yourself for not getting it perfectly right? Are you comparing yourself to others? Practice accepting and loving yourself. Give yourself a big hug, pat yourself on the back, and use positive affirmations such as, "All is well. I love myself. I accept myself. I promise never to say mean things to myself again."

How are we like the cracked pot? Make a list of things we feel are flawed about ourselves. How can we let go of thinking we are inferior? What are our special gifts, and how do they serve others?

How are we like the farmer or the perfect pot? How can we help others, as the farmer did, to find the goodness within? How does perfection make us feel better than others and what problems can this cause? How can we let go of the need for perfection?

Observe things in nature. Observe the diversity. Observe people; notice the differences in clothing, eye color, shape of the nose, texture of the hair. Notice how we are the same, and not the same.

Hug yourself again and repeat, "I am good enough; I have value. All is as it should be."

ASANAS

The pot - Be yourself! Love yourself! Then feel your love and strength as **WARRIOR I**, *virabhadrasana I*. Become the farmer with **WARRIOR III**, *virabhadrasana III*. He's kind and sends out love. Send love to another person with arms extended out in front of you, hands together with index fingers together and pointing out. "Shoot" love to another person in front of you. Traveling along the road use **TRIANGLE**, *trikonasana*. Take a ride down the river with **BOAT POSE**, *navasana*. Create a flower out of a yoga pose. Anything goes! You could try **FEATHER DANCER POSE**, *natarajasana*, or **CAMEL POSE**, *ustrasana*.

MEDITATION AND RELAXATION

Thought watching: Focus on your breath. Notice your thoughts and let them go with the label, "thinking." Come back to your breath and the space that is between the thoughts.

Be aware of any negative thinking by gardening your thoughts, pulling out the "weeds" of negative thoughts. Notice the feeling behind these negative thoughts, and then change the thoughts to something positive. Visualize a shield, or use your arms to fend off negative thoughts the way an action figure fends off villains or bullets. Enjoy the free, happy space within.

Sit with your eyes open, observing what is in front of you. Don't think about what you see, or judge it. Just observe, as if you were a camera, breathe, and feel your body.

TREASURE: Non-Attachment

We desire so many things in this world, and we get very attached to them. We get attached to pleasures, possessions, and thoughts. The rest of the world suffers because of our selfishness. Additionally, by not letting go of our attachments, we are missing the opportunity to discover something new or make a change.

Attachment also is a form of delusion. Notice the dreamlike quality of the world. Things come and go. We can spend our time reaching for things in this world, but they are not the true things we are looking for — the self. The material wonders of the world are beautiful, but they are transitory and conceal the underlying divinity, which is real.

In this story, the monkey is always grasping for something that isn't real; the moon is just a reflection in the water of the real moon above. But the monkey won't let go of his grip, and must persist until, by chance or grace, he is able to pierce his delusion.

THE MONKEY AND THE MOON – Chinese

There was once a monkey happily swinging from tree to tree. He swung to a branch where he saw an amazing sight. Below him was a pond with the glimmering image of the moon shining in the water. He was amazed by its beauty and brilliant white light.

Hanging onto the branch with one paw, he used his other paw to reach for that beautiful moon. He reached and he reached, but no matter how hard he tried, he could not reach the moon. And he refused to let go of the branch to get closer to the moon.

By grace or chance, the branch he was hanging onto broke, and the monkey plunged into the water. He slapped around in the water for a moment, looking for the moon. Then he looked up into the sky and – there! There it was! The monkey saw the moon shining brightly against the dark night's sky.

WORKING WITH THE STORY

ACTIVITIES

Contemplate this story during asana practice, meditation, or relaxation.

Can you name the phases of the moon: new moon, quarter moon, gibbous moon, full moon, and waning moon? The phases, however, are actually an illusion; the sun and the rotation of the earth only make us think the moon has different shapes.

What kinds of things are you attached to? What do you reach after? Being perfect? Material possessions? Looking good? Negative thinking? If you don't get what you want, will you be unhappy or frustrated? Have you tried again and again to achieve something unattainable? Try to let go of one of these attachments. Like the moon dissolving, let it go. Watch it disappear. It may be hard, but don't be a monkey! Sometimes it's necessary to let go to get to the truth.

How do we let go of an attachment? Try turning it around. Instead of saying "I don't like broccoli," say "I like broccoli." Change "I don't like homework" to "I like homework!"

ASANAS

Do the **MOON SALUTATION** *vinyasa* in the asana section of this book.

Contemplate the phases of each pose. In **TRIANGLE**, *trikonasana*, for example, notice the placement of the feet, the hips, the rotation of the trunk, and then finally the extension of the arm. See how a cycle is completed.

MEDITATION AND RELAXATION

Visualize the moon. Make it orange, yellow, or white; full, half, or quarter. Is a cloud floating over it? Allow the moon to dissolve completely and then reappear as something new. Notice this constant flux and be willing to let go as it changes form.

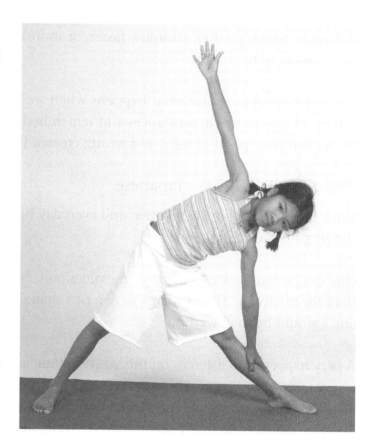

TREASURE: Contentment

"There is nothing either good or bad, but thinking makes it so."
— Shakespeare, *"Hamlet,"* Act 2, Scene 2

In the world, everything just is. Only the mind labels something as good or bad, right or wrong; only the mind makes story and meaning out of existence. If our "doors of perception were cleansed," the world would be as the poet William Blake described it: infinite.

We tend to look at ourselves or things outside ourselves and think that they should be different, newer, prettier, stronger, faster, or more expensive. This causes suffering and a tumultuous state of mine.

This story helps us realize what happens when we are dissatisfied and want to change things. By accepting circumstances and remembering that nothing is wrong with anything except our perception of right and wrong created by the mind, we can find peace within.

THE STONECUTTER – Japanese

Once there was a poor stonecutter, and everyday he went to work at the base of a mountain, slinging his pickaxe into the rock.

One day, when he was exhausted, he said aloud, "Oh, I am just a poor stonecutter, working hard for my living. How I wish I were a rich man. Then all my problems would be solved, and I would be so powerful!"

A fairy happened to listen in on this conversation, and she instantly granted the man his wish.

The poor stonecutter suddenly found that he was a wealthy man. He had delicious food and fine clothes and many servants. Over time, he grew used to this comfortable lifestyle, and with so much power, he began to act bossy and mean.

One day, when the sun was shining harshly and making everybody miserable with its heat, the rich man thought, "Well, this sun has more power than I do. I can't stand it that something has more power than I. I wish I were the sun! Then I would be the most powerful thing in the world!"

The fairy heard the man's wish, and instantly it was granted.

"Haha!" cried the rich man. "Now I am the sun! I am so powerful! I can shine down on everybody, and make their lives great or miserable!" And he blazed his heat down on the poor people below.

His triumph was short-lived, however. Soon a cloud moved in front of the sun and blocked its glaring rays. The sun was furious.

"Why, the cloud is more powerful than I am! I wish to be the cloud so that I can be the most powerful thing in the world!"

Of course, his wish was instantly granted by the nearby fairy. Unfortunately, as a cloud, the rich man was instantly blown away by the wind.

"Oh, no! Make me the wind!" he cried. "The wind is the most powerful thing in the world!" Once again, his wish was granted.

As the wind, the rich man loved blowing over the people, making their lives miserable. He blew all sorts of things: clothes off the line, hats off of heads, roofs off of houses, but he was not satisfied. He couldn't do anything to a mountain that stood before him, tall and unwavering. He blew, and he blew, but his wind had no effect.

"Oh! The mountain is more powerful than I! Make me a mountain!" he cried, and his wish was granted.

As a mountain, the rich man sat beaming with boastful pride at his power and strength. Then, he heard a strange sound.

"Chink, chink, chink," went the sound. "Chink, chink, chink." The mountain thought, "What is that? What is that sound?" He looked down, and there was a poor stonecutter, cutting away at the mountainside.

"Oh, no!" cried the mountain. "That stonecutter is more powerful than I! Eventually, he will cut away the whole mountain! The stonecutter is the most powerful thing in the world! I want to be a stonecutter!" His wish was instantly granted. Once again, he was a poor stonecutter.

WORKING WITH THE STORY

ACTIVITIES

Contemplate this story during asana practice, meditation, or relaxation.

How are you like the stonecutter? What things in your life are you dissatisfied with? Note how it feels to have this dissatisfaction. Make a list of things that you have and enjoy; then make a list of things you want but don't have. How does it feel not to have those things? How can you move your focus from the list of what you don't have, to the list of what you do have?

ASANAS

Try to find contentment in these poses. Notice when you strain your body or try to be perfect; notice when you judge yourself. Stay with your breath and remind yourself that there is nothing wrong. Everything is fine.

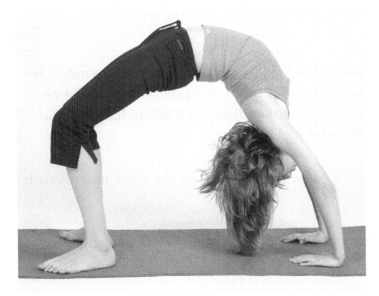

Try a difficult pose, such as **CROW POSE**, *baksasana,* **UPWARD FACING BOW**, *urdva dhanurasana,* **PRETTY POSE**, *rajakapotasana,* **HEADSTAND,** *salamaba sirsasana* or **UNICORN POSE**, *vashistasana.* If you are challenged, remain calm and peaceful. Continue practicing and enjoying the process.

MEDITATION AND RELAXATION

Visualize the mountain, the sun, the cloud, the wind, and the stonecutter. Then visualize things you are dissatisfied with. Afterwards, say silently, "All is well. All is as it should be. Everything is just right for me. I am content. I am at peace."

TREASURE: Self-Study

"Know thyself," Plato tells us. It is essential that we look at ourselves to find the root of our suffering. We tend to blame others, but when we look at that one finger pointing at another, we notice that there are three pointing back at us.

GIFT FROM THE GODS – Hindu

The gods created humans and placed them on the earth. They watched them for many, many years and saw how they used the earth to create wonderful fields, buildings, and tools. They also observed how the humans treated each other.

One day, the gods decided to give the humans a gift.

"You have done very well for yourselves," a god said. "You have learned to make many things from this earth. Well done! We have also noticed where you have not done so well. We have seen you arguing, complaining, and fighting with each other. So we have a gift for you." The gods gave to each human a bag. "In these bags are your faults. We hope you study them well so that you can make your lives even better. That is our gift to you."

But the humans didn't like looking at their bag of faults. Ugh! It was much easier to look into their neighbors' bags and point out *their* faults. So the humans put their own bags of faults on sticks and slung them over their shoulders behind them, where they are carried to this day.

WORKING WITH THE STORY

ACTIVITIES

Contemplate this story during asana practice, meditation, or relaxation.

Make a list of qualities you don't like in others, such as rudeness, bossiness, tardiness, and so on. Afterwards, look at this same list and see if you recognize any of the qualities in yourself.

Pair up with a partner and study each other. Tell your partner what qualities you see in him. For instance, you may say, "You have kind eyes. You seem to be a smart person. I sense you are a little bit worried." Be careful to be kind and not overly critical. Now switch places.

ASANA

Video tape the class doing asana practice. During this session, try some difficult poses, such as **UNICORN POSE**, *vashistasana*, **CROW POSE**, *bakasana*, or **HALF MOON POSE**, *ardha chandrasana*. You may fall over when you first attempt these asanas, but be gentle with yourself when you see yourself on video.

MEDITATION AND RELAXATION

Visualize a bag that is a gift from the gods. Inside your bag are the qualities you need to improve within yourself. What are they? Paying attention? Being more kind? Say to the imaginary gods, "Thank you for this knowledge of my faults. I am getting better every day." Now visualize your best qualities. Say to the imaginary gods, "Thank you for this knowledge of my talents. I know that I am very special."

TREASURE: Surrender

Mythologist Joseph Campbell says that we should stop living the life we think we want and start living the life that is waiting for us. In other words, "Let go and let God." This is essential if we want to live a peaceful life. By surrendering, we find what we are looking for, and it's greater than what we can imagine. Just like in fairy tales, in life, you get what you want, just not in the way you expected to get it.

THE STORY OF THE SANDS – Sufi

A river was making its way down from a mountain top toward the great sea below. Guided by a voice from within, it moved over the rocky face of the mountain toward its destiny.

Suddenly, it came upon a great desert. No matter how hard the river pushed, its water was absorbed into the sand, and the journey halted. The river did not know what to do. So, it continued the only way it knew, pushing and pushing and pushing. Finally, exhausted and frustrated, the river gave up.

Suddenly, an overhead cloud spoke. "River, I know of your desire to reach the sea. That is your destiny. But you cannot cross the sand."

"Yes, I know," said the river, and it struggled one last time against the sand before giving up.

"I will help you," said the cloud. "Let yourself be absorbed into me. I will take you to your destination."

But the little river resisted. It was afraid. Absorb itself into the cloud? It had never done anything like that before.

"Trust me, little river, I can help you," the cloud said. "There is nothing to fear."

The little river sat for a while, exhausted. It gave one last push, and then collapsed.

"OK, I will trust you," the river said.

Drop by drop, the river was lifted up, up, up through the air and into the cloud. The cloud grew heavy and dark as it absorbed the little river.

Being part of the cloud, the river wasn't afraid. In fact, it felt like it was remembering something familiar and peaceful.

The cloud carried the river over the great desert. Then, in a great burst of thunder and a streak of lightning, the cloud released the river into millions of little drops of water that poured down beyond the desert, and the river became itself again, rapidly moving once again toward the sea.

WORKING WITH THE STORY

ACTIVITIES

Contemplate this story during asana practice, meditation, or relaxation. How are you like the river? Are you afraid to let go of something? Are you trying to force the result of something? Find examples in your life where you surrendered and things worked out for the better.

ASANA

Let go during this practice: do not force anything or focus on a specific result. **SEATED FORWARD BEND,** *pashimotanasana*, is a good pose for surrender. Add poses as desired such as **HERO,** *virasana*. Take more time for relaxation with the **CORPSE POSE,** *shavasana*, to let go.

MEDITATION AND RELAXATION

Imagine yourself walking down a forest path. You'll come to a cliff that overlooks a beautiful canyon. Down below is the unknown. Jump off the cliff. Let go, and fall freely, fearlessly. Down, down you'll go, until you feel yourself landing gently on your feet.

Now imagine yourself on a huge wave. The wave is tossing and turning you. The wave finally comes to rest with you on the shore, safe and sound.

Visualize a door on the side of a great oak tree and enter it. Inside is a huge well. Dive into that well and drop down, down, down. Feel the falling, but trust that all will be all right. An adventure awaits you. What is it?

TREASURE: Courage

The word courage comes from the Latin root *"cor,"* which means heart. When we have courage, we are living from the heart. This heart is as strong and fearless as a lion. It feels fear only when the mind creates a false belief of separation from others or the environment.

THE THREE SISTERS - Muslim

Every year Disease makes a visit to the holy city of Mecca. Her companions are always her sisters Death and Fear. One year, Fear went ahead of Death and Disease. The old gatekeeper, who did not know Fear, let her go into the city.

When Death and Disease arrived at the gate of Mecca, the gatekeeper called out angrily, "So, Disease, you've come again to bring Death and misery to people! How many victims will you take this time?"

"No more than 500 I'm sure," Disease said.

"Ok," said the gatekeeper. "Promise not to take any more! And you, Death, how many will you take?"

"Oh, I will take what Disease gives me."

The gatekeeper let them by, warning then not to take more than they promised.

Weeks later, Death and Disease returned and called to the gatekeeper to open the gate.

"Well, Disease, how many did you take?" the gatekeeper asked.

"Oh, I took only 499," Disease said.

"Any you, Death, how many did you take?" the gatekeeper asked.

"Oh, I took more than a thousand."

"But you promised that you'd only take what Disease gave you!" the gatekeeper cried.

"Yes," Death answered, "But most of those who died were taken by our sister Fear, who went unnoticed through your gate. One day, you will know, old man, that our sister Fear does more harm and causes more death than Disease!"

WORKING WITH THE STORY

ACTIVITIES

Contemplate this story during asana, meditation, and relaxation.

Take out your journal and write about your fears. Can you think back to any event in your life that made you afraid? Retell that story.

What can we do if we are afraid? Who can we talk to? Many times we are afraid to do things because we want to look good. Is fear a choice?

ASANAS

Practice grounding poses, such as **WARRIOR I, II** and **III,** *virabhradrasana I, II, III.* Focus on the feet, legs and hips. Try **PIGEON POSE**, *eka pada rajakapotanasana* and **BOUND ANGLE POSE**, *badhha konasana.* Let the lower half of the body come into awareness. Imagine the energy flowing from the heart, through the body, down to the hips, to the toes, then flowing out and connecting to the universe. Feel the energy of the body flowing to the floor and to the people in the room. Feel the connection and support of the universe. There is no need to be afraid. Everything is part of you.

Also practice heart opening poses, such as **CAMEL POSE**, *ustrasana*, **COBRA POSE**, *bhujangasana*, **UPWARD FACING BOW POSE**, *urdva dhanurasana*, **FISH POSE**, *matsyasana*, and **BOW POSE**, *dhanurasana*.

Try **SHOULDERSTAND**, *salamba sharvangasana*. At first, this may feel frightening. Take small steps toward the pose, even if it's just taking the formation of the pose, or being in bridge pose, or rocking.

Try **LION POSE**, *simhasana*. Roar and feel courageous!

MEDITATION AND RELAXATION

Become aware of your body. Focus on each body part and how it feels connected to other body parts. Become aware of energy, pain, and tension in your body. Now think of something that makes you afraid and talk to that feeling. Tell it that you understand what it's going through. What does the fear say back?

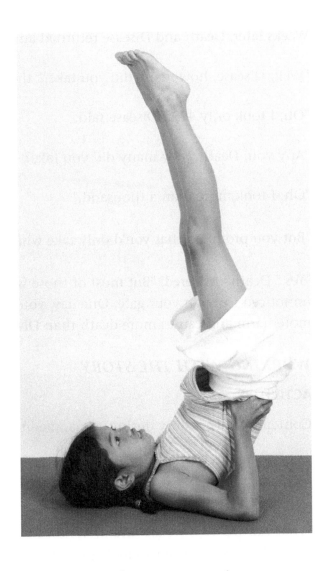

Visualize something that scares you, and replace that image with a courageous image. Mentally create a badge of courage. Decorate it with your imagination, and afterwards, create the badge with art materials.

CALMING THE STORM – Christian

One day the twelve disciples and Jesus got into a boat on the sea. Jesus quickly fell asleep in the rocking waves. But soon, a terrible storm swept up, tossing the boat to and fro. The twelve disciples were terrified.

"Master, Master!" they cried. "Please, wake up! We are afraid! We will drown in this storm!"

Jesus woke up. He stood up and said, "Oh, ye of little faith." He looked out on the storm, stretched out his hands and said, "Peace." Instantly, the storm calmed. All was well once again.

WORKING WITH THE STORY

ACTIVITIES

Contemplate this story during asana, relaxation, or meditation.

When you are feeling afraid, focus on slow, deep, rhythmic breathing. Put your hand on your belly, and let the belly be pushed out by the breathing. What does the belly say? What is it afraid of? What do you say to it? Is it true? Is it happening right now? Or is it an if?

ASANA

Fear can be dealt with by developing a strong core and trust in the Self. These poses develop a strong core. Start with **BOAT POSE**, *navasana*. Then lower down into **HALF BOAT**, *ardha navasana*. Finish up with **KNEE TO HEAD POSE**.

MEDITATION AND RELAXATION

Loving-kindness practice is an antidote for fear. Replace fearful thoughts with those of love and kindness. During difficult times, practice this mantra for five minutes each day: "May I find freedom from fear. May I help others be free from fear."

TREASURE: Stillness

He that does nothing does everything, says the *Tao Te Ching*.

Often, we are trying to get something or to get away from something. Such desire and aversion pulls us from our place of peaceful stillness into the world, and this causes suffering. Of course, we will always have desires and aversions, but we can temper the way they affect us. When we feel sad, we can cry, and when we are happy, we can be happy, but we need to understand that these states are impermanent; we can always return to our state of peaceful stillness.

STANDING STILL – Jewish

One day, when the Rabbi was in the marketplace watching all the people rushing to and fro, he grabbed one man's arm and held him.

"Hey!" the man cried, trying to pull away. "What do you think you are doing? Let me go! I have important things to do, places to see! Things to get!"

The Rabbi held fast to the man's arm and said, "How do you know that what you are looking for is in front of you? Maybe what you are looking for is behind you, and all you have to do is stand still until it all catches up with you."

WORKING WITH THE STORY

ACTIVITIES

Contemplate this story during asana practice, meditation, or relaxation.

Make a list of all the things you do in your life. Is it a lot or a little? Do you feel rushed? Does one part of your body feel rushed? Touch that part of your body and talk to it. What does it say? What is really important? How can you take time to slow down and enjoy things more?

ASANA

Try a resting pose, such as **CHILD'S POSE**, *balasana*, and a restorative pose, such as **SHOULDER STAND**, *salamba sharvangasana*. Try to hold the poses for a long period of time before moving into **PLOW POSE**, *halasana*. Try holding other poses longer.

MEDITATION AND RELAXATION

There is nothing to do; there is nothing to get, nowhere to go, nothing to buy or compete for. Just BE. For now, release yourself from the need to DO. Create an image of this relaxing, free feeling. Afterwards, draw the image.

THE HEART THAT NO LONGER MOVES – Sufi

One day the servant of a prosperous merchant came bursting through the master's door.

"Master! Master!" he cried. "I have terrible news! Our ship carrying much merchandise was lost at sea! Our fortune is lost! We are ruined!"

The Master stood still, looked down at his heart, and said, *"Allah Akbara"* (God is great). Then he said, "Thank you for this news."

The servant went away, only to come back the next day crying, "Master! Master!" Jumping up and down, he said, "Master, I have great news! It was a mistake! The ship wasn't lost after all! It was someone else's ship! We are saved! We still have all our wealth!"

The Master again, stood still, looked down at his heart, and said, *"Allah Akbara."*

The servant looked at his Master strangely. "Master, I do not understand. Every time I say something, whether it is good or bad news, you just look down. What is that all about?"

"Ah," the Master said. "Each time I was looking down at my heart to make sure that it did not move."

WORKING WITH THE STORY

ACTIVITIES

Contemplate this story during asana practice, meditation, or relaxation.

Make a list of things you like. Select a few of these items; if you have the item, how does it feel? How does it feel if you don't have the item?

Return to the breath and notice how the breath feels cold when it comes in the nose and hot when it leaves the nose. Be still and ask yourself, who is observing my breath? Who is the "I" watching these thoughts and this action? Notice how easily this "I" accepts the cold and the hot.

ASANA

Practice the **STAFF OF BRAHMA** *vinyasa*. Become aware of your breath, body, and movement. Find a still point in each moment, even during movement. With each breath and movement, reinforce the idea that there is stillness, a still, one-pointed awareness.

MEDITATION AND RELAXATION

Visualize a sun with wings on each side of it. Focus on the singularity of the sun, duality of movement, and the world in the wings.

TREASURE: Sacrifice

Sacrifice means to make something sacred, to perform a priestly duty, and to give something up for something or someone else. All of life is a sacrifice: animals and plants give up their lives to feed humans or return to the earth to feed other plants and animals. Parents sacrifice their time and money to raise children. In Dionysian and Christian myth, something is shattered and sacrificed so that something new can be made.

In this story we learn about what it means to give something up and how it serves the world.

THE SPIRIT WHO LIVED IN A TREE - Buddhist

The Buddha decided to become a tree. He became a Sal tree and grew for sixty thousand years. Beneath the tree's enormous branches, hundreds of little Sal trees grew as well. This tree was so enormous and beautiful that all of the people in the nearby village would come and worship it. The King of Benares soon heard of the great tree.

"Some kings have their palaces built with many pillars. Well, I shall build my palace with only one great pillar in the middle. This Sal tree shall be that pillar. I order it cut down!"

All of the townspeople were dismayed. They loved the tree, but they were too frightened not to carry out the King's orders.

One night, the people lit oil lamps and walked to the great tree. They tied a nosegay of flowers around its trunk. Then they prayed, "Oh, Great Spirit that resides in this tree, the King has ordered that in seven days, we must cut you down. We don't want to do it, but we fear for our families. Please spirit, go somewhere else, and do no harm to us. Forgive us. We love you, and we will miss you greatly."

The tree spirit thought, *this King is determined to cut me down, but my life only lasts as long as this tree. The thought of my death does not bother me as much as ….ah! Look at the little Sal trees around me! Their death and destruction is more painful to me than my own death.*

So that night, at midnight, a bright golden light filled the King's room, and the tree spirit appeared next to the King's bed, weeping.

The King awoke. "Oh! Who are you spirit, and why have you come? Why do you weep?"

"I am the spirit that lives in the tree you wish to cut down. I ask that you spare my life."

The King thought a moment. "No, I cannot. I want my palace to stand on only one tree, and you will be that tree. I must cut you down."

"Then please," said the spirit, "I make one request."

"What is that?" the King asked.

"Please cut me down bit by bit. Begin with the branches; then cut the trunk; and cut down to the roots last of all."

"Why, this is a most painful death," the King said. "One swift blow at the roots would fell you, and you would be out of your misery."

The spirit said, "Yes, it is painful. But it is not as painful as seeing the beloved little Sal trees around me destroyed by my fall. Please, I ask you to honor my request."

The King was deeply moved by the tree's spirit of sacrifice.

"Oh, spirit," the King said, "Fear not. Your great concern for the life of others has moved me deeply. I will not cut you down. Return, great tree, to the forest in peace."

WORKING WITH THE STORY

ACTIVITIES

Contemplate this story during asana practice, meditation, or relaxation.

Write down how you are like the tree. What have you given up for somebody else? Can you give your food, time, or money, or do you have a special talent to share, such as playing a musical instrument at a nursing home?

Are you holding onto a grudge? If so, can you sacrifice the need to be right or the need to punish? Can you find forgiveness and make peace?

Take a walk among trees. Draw trees. Make a collage of pressed leaves.

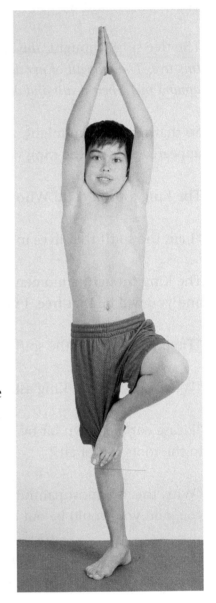

ASANAS

TREE POSE, *vrksasana*. Contemplate yourself as a tree, firmly rooted in the earth but reaching for the heavens. Imagine that energy flows through your trunk. Roots run down your legs deep into the earth. Your arms are limbs reaching to the sky where your fingers flower with their unique gifts. Imagine the energy of the tree. Recall how still trees are. By being still, we conserve and focus our energy. We are powerful!

Move from **TREE POSE**, *vrksasana*, to **WARRIOR III**, *virabhradrasana III*, in one swoop. Do both sides.

Use **SHOULDERSTAND**, *salamba sharvangasana*, to imagine that the tree is reversed and your wiggling toes are the roots.

MEDITATION AND RELAXATION

Visualize a tree inside your heart. Breathing in, the tree branches spread through the upper part of your body. Breathing out, the roots sink deep into the earth. What do you want in the world? What is your greatest desire? Visualize these things as blossoms on your limbs. Then let them fall to the ground. Imagine them gone. Consider the sacred nature of sacrifice.

TREASURE: Compassion

"Mercy is setting the prisoner free, only to discover the prisoner was me."
– Anonymous

When we have compassion for others, we have compassion for ourselves.

THE BANYAN DEER – Buddhist

Long ago, the Bodhisat took a life as King of the Banyan deer. He was a radiant color of gold, with eyes like round jewels; his horns glimmered like silver. His mouth was as red as a rose; his hooves were bright and hard like lacquer work; his tail was fine, and his body large.

The King of the Banyan Deer lived in the forest with a herd of 500 attendant deer. Not far away lived another deer as golden as he, and he was called the King of the Monkey Deer and had a big herd as well.

Now, the human king of this country loved to hunt and never ate a single meal without meat. Every day, he summoned the townspeople to accompany him hunting, whether they wanted to or not. Soon, the people began to complain.

"This King with his insistent hunting practices puts an end to our work, and I never get anything done," one townsperson cried.

"Yes, I'm tired of this!" another one said. "Let's just make a park. We'll provide food and drink for the deer, drive them in, and then close the entrance. The King can go in there and hunt all he wants, and we won't have to disrupt our schedules anymore."

So that's what the townspeople did, surrounding the very place where the Monkey Deer and the Banyan Deer were living. The King was excited to go to the park and hunt, and when he got there, he saw the two remarkable golden deer.

"What fabulous creatures you are!" he cried. I grant you your lives." And he went to shoot another deer and brought it home.

Sometimes the King's cook would go and shoot a deer. The deer, as soon as they saw his bow and arrow, would shake with fear of death and run away. The cook, however, wasn't a very good shot, and when he pursued the deer, they would get wounded and become weary. The herd told their King, and he sent for the King of the Monkey Deer.

"Friend, the deer are being destroyed. All things must die; however, let them not be wounded with arrows," the King of the Banyan Deer said. "Let the deer take turns at a place of execution. One day the lot can fall on my herd, and the next on yours." So every day, one deer lay down and placed his neck on a chopping block, and the cook came and carried off the one he found lying there.

One day, the lot fell on a doe that was heavy with young. She went to the King of the Monkey Deer and cried, "Please! I am with young! After I have brought forth my baby, we shall both take our turn on the block. Please order the lot to pass me by."

But the King of the Monkey Deer refused. So she turned to the King of the Banyan Deer and pleaded with him. The Bodhisat listened quietly and said. "So be it. Go back. I will relieve you of your turn." And he himself went to lay his head on the chopping block at the place of execution.

The cook, seeing him, ran back to the King and said, "The King of the Deer whose life you promised to him is lying in the place of execution. What does it mean?"

Baffled, the King mounted his chariot and road out to the park. Seeing the Bodisat, he said, "Friend! King of the Deer! I granted you your life! Why are you lying here?"

"Oh, great King!" The Bodhisat said. "A doe heavy with young came to me. The lot had fallen upon her to be taken. I could not ask another to take her place, so I took it instead. Have no more suspicion, great King!"

"Ah, you golden-colored King of the Deer," the king exclaimed. "Never before have I seen such mercy, kindness, and compassion. I am pleased with you in this matter! Rise up. I grant life to you and the doe!"

"Although we are safe," the Bodhisat said, "what about the other deer in the park?"

"I grant them their lives, my Lord," the King said.

"But what of the other animals in the forest — the birds in the sky, the fish in the streams — how will they obtain peace?"

"I grant all birds, fish, and animals their lives. None shall hunt them," the King declared.

Having interceded with the King for all creatures, the great being said, "Walk in righteousness, O great King! By doing justice and mercy to fathers and mothers, to sons and daughters, to townsmen and landsmen, when your body is dissolved, you shall enter the happy world of heaven!"

WORKING WITH THE STORY

ACTIVITIES

Contemplate this story during asana practice, meditation, or relaxation.

How are we like the King, wanting things and ordering people to do what we want? How can we help others? Sometimes there are rules in our society that prevent us from doing a compassionate act, in the same way that the Monkey Deer could not help the mother doe. What would you do in such a situation? How are we like the King of the Banyan Deer? What things have we done for others who needed our help?

How are our thoughts and speech like "arrows" that can wound others? Think of someone that you don't like. Notice how you feel thinking about this person. Our thoughts have energy to disrupt ourselves and also cause unease in the world. Notice the negative feeling and shift it into one of love for the person you don't like, and set them "free." How do you feel after sending the person love? Next time you are around that person, continue sending thoughts of love. See if that relationship changes over time.

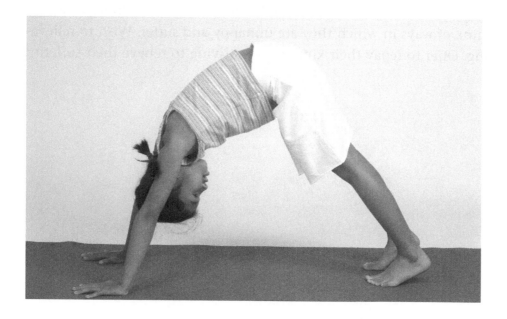

ASANA

Be the King and take **WARRIOR I**, *virabhadrasana I*. Then become the King of the Banyan Deer with **WARRIOR II**, *virabhadrasana II* and the Monkey King with **DOWNWARD DOG**, *adho mukha svanasana*. Travel with **TRIANGLE**, *trikonasana*, in the forest **TREE POSE**, *vrksasana*. Become the Cook with **FEATHER DANCER POSE**, *natarajasana*. The Doe as **PIGEON POSE**, *eka pada rajakapotasana prep*. Make the Chopping Block as **BOUND ANGLE POSE**, *baddha konasana*. The King's heart opens when he realizes the truth. Try **CAMEL POSE**, *ustrasana*. Add additional asanas of backbends and heart opening poses, such as **BRIDGE POSE**, *setu bandha sharvangasana*, **BOW POSE**, *dhanurasana*, and **COBRA POSE**, *bhujangasana*. Lie with a bolster under your shoulders and breath and to let the natural effect of gravity open the heart.

MEDITATION AND RELAXATION

Focus on the heart center and repeat silently to the sound of "Yum."

Drop your attention to your heart center and listen as characters from the story are called out: Banyan Deer, Monkey Deer, King, Cook. Imagine each character when you hear the name, and send feelings of love and mercy toward that character. Now, think of somebody you don't like and send love, mercy, and compassion toward him or her.

Compassion Meditation: Think of people in this order: first the parent it's easiest for you to get along with, then the second parent, then a distant relative, then a stranger. Now think about "enemies" or people you have a troubled relationship with. Visualize each person clearly. Remember what acts of kindness they have done. Wish to repay their kindness. Think of ways in which they are unhappy and suffer. Wish to relieve them of their suffering. Offer to repay their kindness by striving to relieve their suffering.

TREASURE: Kindness

The golden rule, *Do unto others as you would have done unto you*, is found in twenty-one religions. Everything that goes from you comes back to you. If you are kind and peaceful, kindness and peace comes back to you.

MOHAMMAD AND THE CAT – Muslim

One morning, many pupils gathered around the great prophet Mohammad to hear his teaching. As he began to teach in the early morning rays of the sun, a little cat came and curled up next to him on the tail of his robe and fell asleep.

The prophet continued teaching as the sun rose high in the sky. At noon, the little cat was still asleep on his robe. The prophet continued teaching as the sun began to lower behind the mountains in the afternoon, and the little cat went on sleeping.

After the lesson was over, the students left. The cat still slept. Mohammad looked at the little cat still sleeping on his robe. He reached for the dagger he kept by his side, and as carefully as possible, he cut the fabric of his cloak in order to free himself without disturbing the sleeping cat.

WORKING WITH THE STORY

ACTIVITIES

Contemplate this story during asana, relaxation, or meditation.

What is kindness? How can we be kind? For example, can we hold the door open for some-one, or carry groceries for the elderly? What kinds of animals are in our lives? What about the animals we eat? Should we treat them with kindness as well? How? Let's talk about the importance of humane conditions for animals that we eat. Can we be kind to the earth? Let's talk about organic food and the environment.

ASANA

Have fun with animal poses: **EAGLE POSE**, *garudasana*, **FISH POSE**, *matsyasana*, **RABBIT POSE**, *sasangasana*, and **CAT POSE**, *bidalasana*. Try **DOWNWARD DOG**, *adho mukha svanasana*, and **PIGEON POSE**, *eka pada rajakapotanasana*.

TREASURE: Controlling the Mind

The Yoga Sutra 1.2 says, *Chitta Vritti Narodaha*, or *Yoga is the cessation of the fluctuations of the mind*. The mind is continually creating stories about life, playing tricks on us, causing fears and desires and delusion. Yoga gives us the discipline we need to find the clarity of our true selves.

PRAYING THE PSALMS – Jewish

There was once a young woman who was sweeping out her parents' house. She sang to herself in delight as she dreamt of the man she would one day marry.

"Oh, we will have a wonderful wedding!" she thought. "How happy we will be! And we will have a lovely child. He will be so adorable and sweet!" But then her mood changed. She stopped sweeping. "Oh! But what if my baby should get sick as an infant! What if he should die? Oh, this would be terrible!" And she began sobbing hysterically.

Her parents rushed in. "What is wrong, dear child?"

The daughter explained her sad story about what could happen. Her parents, swayed by the sadness, also began crying hysterically. The neighbors stopped by and inquired what was wrong. When they heard the story, they broke out sobbing. Soon all of the townspeople were inside the house crying terribly over the fate of this young girl.

The Rabbi stopped by, asked what was happening, and replied. "There is only one thing to do; we must pray the Psalms." And with that, he opened his book.

Now a baker, who was not from the town, stopped by and wondered what was going on. When he found out what they were crying about, he said, "HOLD ON! Everything you are upset about is based on IFS. IF you get married, IF you have a son, IF he gets sick, and IF he dies. None of it has happened at all! It's not real!"

Everyone stared quietly at the baker for a moment, then burst out laughing, and all was well again.

"You see," the Rabbi said, "that's what happens when you pray the Psalms."

WORKING WITH THE STORY

ACTIVITIES

Contemplate this story during asana practice, meditation, or relaxation.

What are some of your "Ifs"? If I don't pass this test, if my friend doesn't like me, if I lose my bike... Although the "Ifs" may seem real, they are nothing but thoughts. We can use the breath to bring us back to reality, where anything that does happen to us can be dealt with clearly in the present moment.

WALKING ON WATER – Christian

An archbishop was on a voyage when he saw three figures on an apparently deserted island. He wanted to convert them to Christianity, so he had a small boat bring him to shore.

When the three men saw a holy man approaching, they immediately bowed down.

Surprised, the archbishop said, "Are you men Christians?"

"We pray to be," one said. "But we are hermits, and have been here so long that we have forgotten what to do or what to say."

"Well, then show me how you pray," the archbishop said.

The men began to pray: "Lord, have mercy on sinners such as we..."

"Stop, stop!" the archbishop shouted. "Goodness, don't you know the Lord's Prayer?"

"We don't remember it," they said. "Please, do teach it to us."

So the archbishop went over the Lord's Prayer, starting with "Our Father, who art in heaven." He said it, thinking they would understand such a simple and short prayer quickly.

But this was not the case. The men needed to go over it several times; they asked questions; and it took the entire day before they learned it.

His work done, the archbishop went back to his boat and pushed off, noting that the three men were still practicing the prayer he had taught them so well.

The next day, the archbishop stood on the ship looking out over the horizon. The island he had left was out of sight, but he could faintly make out in the mist three figures coming toward him from the direction of the island. He looked harder into the mist, and was amazed at what he saw. Sure enough, it was the three hermits from the island, running on the water toward him!

"Your Grace," they cried out. "We have forgotten the prayer. Please do not be angry with us, but please do teach it to us again!"

"Go in peace my friends," the archbishop said humbly. "Go and pray the way you have been. It is fine." So they did.

WORKING WITH THE STORY

ACTIVITIES

Contemplate this story during asana practice, meditation, or relaxation.

Talk about how many ways there are to do one thing: eating, sleeping, praying, working, playing, exercising. The universe is unlimited. Trillions of universes and stars are out there. Is there only one way life or a planet could be? Why or why not? How can our thoughts limit our lives? How does imposing our thoughts on others cause problems?

HEAVEN AND HELL – Zen

There was once a great Samurai, who went to see a Master teacher to learn more. He came before the teacher and said, "Master, I would like to know if heaven and hell exist."

The teacher heard this and burst out laughing. "You silly fool! You would like to know about heaven and hell? Just look at you. You're an uneducated slob. I will not teach somebody like you." And the Master turned his back on the Samurai.

The Samurai's face flushed red with anger. Breathing heavily, he drew his sword and was about to chop off the Master's head when the Master turned around and calmly said, "That, sir, is hell."

The Samurai stopped in his tracks and realized the truth in the Master's teachings. He saw immediately how he created his own hell with his pride and anger. He dropped the sword and fell to his knees, weeping in humble reverence.

"Master, forgive me," the Samurai said.

The master looked down at him, lifted his head, and said, "And that, sir, is heaven."

WORKING WITH THE STORY

ACTIVITIES

Contemplate this story during asana practice, meditation, or relaxation.

Notice how your thoughts can affect your feelings in the body. When you are angry or joyous, how does it feel? Can you choose how you want to feel? Talk about times in your life when you were in "heaven" or in "hell."

TREASURE: Anger Control

To be peaceful, we must get in control of our emotions. Anger is a difficult one to master, but we can remember that it is a secondary emotion. People, places, and things remind us of something that is still wounded within us, and we lash out with anger to defend our softness. Next time you get angry, ask yourself, what is this really about? Are you humiliated, made wrong, offended? Instead of reacting in anger, take time to cool down and think about what happened. Talk about it. Meditate, practice some asanas, and try to be in the moment.

THE LOTUS ON THE ROOF – Hindu

Once, there was a couple who practiced yoga regularly. Their health was excellent, abundance overflowed in their household, and the whole town loved them. Their next-door neighbors, however, were intensely jealous; anger burned in their hearts. One day, the neighbor man decided to do something about it.

"I want you to burn down their house!" he cried to a bad man who was paid to do such things.

"Agreed, but how will I know which house to burn down?" the bad man asked.

"I will put a lotus on the roof."

That night, the jealous neighbor brought home a lotus. His wife saw it and said, "Oh! What a lovely lotus! Is it for me?"

"No," her husband snapped. He put it on the neighbors' roof and went to sleep.

But the wife couldn't sleep. "Why should my neighbors have such a beautiful lotus and not me? I deserve it!"

So she climbed out of bed, took the lotus off the neighbors' roof and put it on theirs. And their house burned down instead.

WORKING WITH THE STORY

ACTIVITIES

Contemplate this story during asana practice, meditation, or relaxation.
How do our emotions affect us? Was there a time when you felt jealous of another person? What happened? What can we do to appreciate what we have and not want what others have? How does anger and jealousy "burn down our own house?".

ASANAS

HALF LOTUS POSE, *ardha padmasana*. Notice your body and where there may be tension, pain, or another sensation try **FULL LOTUS,** *padmasana*.

Think of something that makes you very angry. Sit with the anger and ask, what is the feeling behind the anger? Is it humiliation? Sadness? Frustration? Fear? Thich Nhat Hahn says that when we bring mindfulness to our anger, it will slowly disappear.

THE BROKEN MIRRORS — Hindu

Once there was a poor man who had a big bag of mirrors. One day while he was walking to the market to sell the mirrors, he set the bag down to rest. As he rested, he began to think.

"I'm going to sell all these mirrors in the market today! Just think, I will be able to buy even more mirrors with the profits, and then I can buy and sell more mirrors! Eventually, I will be so wealthy! I will be able to ask for the hand of a princess! Why, she will live happily with me!"

But then the man thought of something else. "Well! What if she isn't happy? What if she starts to complain, or wants something else?" He began to get angry. "Ha! If ever she should get angry with me or not agree with me, why, I'll put a stop to that in a hurry!"

He took his foot and kicked the bag forcefully, shattering all the mirrors inside. And that was the end of his plans.

WORKING WITH THE STORY

ACTIVITIES

Contemplate this story during asana practice, meditation, or relaxation.

How do this man's dreams compare with his reality? Were his dreams reachable? How do his fantasies affect his reality?

Compare your life with this story. When have you fantasized about something? Did it come true? If it did come true, did it turn out the way you expected? If not, why not?

ASANA

If you are feeling angry, practice your favorite asanas to help move the energy.

CONEJITO and the WAX DOLL – Yaqui/Zapotec

Once there was a little rabbit, *un Conejito*, and he loved to go into the farmer's garden, *el huerto*, and eat the chilies, *los chiles*; the carrots, *las zanahorias*; and the cucumbers, *los pepinos*.

Each the morning, the farmer would see *Conejito's* footprints and get angry that he ate his crops. So the farmer came up with a trick. He made a large doll out of wax and stuck it in the middle of the garden.

At midnight under a full moon, *Conejito* came back to the garden. He saw the wax doll. "Hola," he said. "*¿Cómo estás?*" How are you?" The wax doll said nothing.

"I said, *Hola*," *Conejito* said again. "How are you? Why don't you answer me?" Still there was no answer. "Do you think that you are better than me? Is that why you won't talk to me?" Still, no answer came from the wax doll.

"Well!" *Conejito* started to get angry. "Let me tell you something then!" *Conejito* took his right fist and punched the wax doll. But his fist stuck in the wax, and no matter how hard he tried, he couldn't pull his fist free.

As he got even angrier, *Conejito's* face turned red. He hit the doll with his left fist. Now both fists were stuck in the wax. He got even angrier, and kicked the wax doll with his right foot. That got stuck too! He got more and more angry and kicked the doll with his left foot. Now *Conejito* was really stuck.

In the morning, the farmer came to his field again. There was *Conejito*, stuck to the doll. The farmer pulled *Conejito* off the doll, stuffed him into a bag, and took him home where he started to boil a big pot of water for lunch.

WORKING WITH THE STORY

ACTIVITIES

Contemplate this story during asana practice, meditation, or relaxation.

Ask children, how does reacting to anger with physical violence get us "stuck?" *Conejito* made up a "story" when the wax doll did not answer. Was it true? How does assuming things about others get us into trouble? What alternatives could we imagine instead of fighting to resolve the problem? Make up alternative endings to the story.

ASANA

Add yoga poses to the story, such as the **RABBIT POSE**, *sasangasana*. Use the **BOAT POSE**, *navasana*, without straightening your legs for when *Conejito* is stuck on the wax doll.

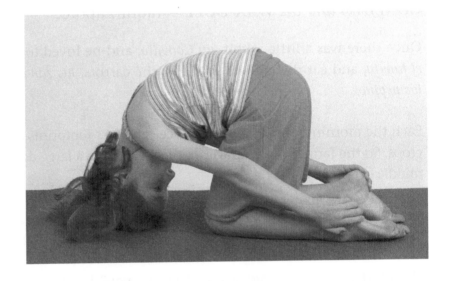

THE TWO WOLVES – Cherokee

There was once an old Cherokee who was teaching his grandson about life. "You know, there is a terrible fight going on inside me," he said to the boy. "This fight is between two wolves. One of these wolves is evil — he is anger, envy, sorrow, regret, greed, arrogance, self-pity, guilt, resentment, inferiority, deceit, false pride, superiority, and ego. The other wolf is good — he is joy, peace, love, hope, serenity, humility, kindness, benevolence, empathy, generosity, truth, compassion, and faith."

"Is it going on inside of me, too, grandfather?" the boy asked.

"Yes, it is, and inside every other person, too."

"Which wolf is going to win?" the boy asked.

"The one you feed," the old Cherokee replied.

WORKING WITH THE STORY

ACTIVITIES

Contemplate this story during asana practice, meditation, or relaxation.

Where is your attention? Is it on the evil wolf and its qualities? Or the good wolf? What can you do to transform yourself into a different world?

ASANA

Wolves – **DOWNWARD FACING DOG**, *adho mukha svanasana*. Act out the emotions of the evil and good wolf.

MEDITATION AND RELAXATION

If you are upset and angry right now, forget meditation and relaxation. Take a brisk walk, do more yoga, or dance. Get the energy moving through and out of your body.

TREASURE: Gratitude

Everything in our life has value. Even if disaster strikes, we may be grateful for our strength to persevere, to help another, or to find new talents within us. This story helps us to remember that no matter what happens in our life, we can choose to make something good out of it. Instead of plunging into despair, we can maintain balance and calm and see goodness in everything.

THE CHERRY BLOSSOMS – Zen

The nun Rengetsu was returning from a pilgrimage when she stopped in a town to rest for the night. Although she appeared tired and hungry, each door she knocked on refused her lodging. As the sun began to set behind the hills, she hiked up to a cherry orchard on the hillside. There she made a little bed of leaves under the trees and fell asleep.

But something stirred her in the middle of the night. A beautiful scent fell over her. Pulling herself up from sleep, she beheld the loveliest of sights — the black sky behind dozens of trees with pink cherry blossoms, all blooming radiant and shimmering in the moonlight.

Rengetsu took in the beautiful experience. Then she turned toward the town, gave a little bow, and said, "Oh, people of the village, thank you so much for turning me away tonight. For if you did receive me, then I would never have been able to witness such beauty."

WORKING WITH THE STORY

ACTIVITIES

Contemplate this story during asana practice, meditation, or relaxation.

Make a list of things you are grateful for and read it daily. Write a story about something difficult that happened and how you dealt with it. Identify what talent or strength came out of this experience.

ASANA

Be the nun on your journey of life with **WARRIOR I**, *virabhradrasana I*, Travel up the hill with **TRIANGLE**, *trikonasana*, and among the trees **TREE POSE**, *vrksasana*, take a rest in **SEATED TWIST**, *ardha matsyendrasana* and **FISH POSE**, *matsyasana*. See the beautiful moon **HALF MOON POSE**, *ardha chandrasana*.

MEDITATION AND RELAXATION

Breath in "yes" to your life with gratitude. As you exhale, envision sending that gratitude out to the universe. Inhaling, say "yes," and know that the gratitude is coming back to you in the form of love and abundance.

TREASURE: The Eternal Cycle

In life, all things complete a cycle. From the death of winter is born the life of spring. Energy cannot be destroyed; it just changes form. A snake sheds his old skin to grow a new one, and even stars die and are born again in new forms. There is no need to fear death because we are children of God, part of the eternal cycle.

CHILDREN OF WAX – Africa

There was once a man and a woman who were very happily married, except for one thing. They did not have any children. Day in and day out, they prayed for children. One day the gods decided to answer their prayers and give them children, but these children had one very special feature. They were made of wax.

Because the sun was so hot outside, the children of wax could not go out and work during the day like all the other children who helped their parents. They had to stay inside all day, but when the hot sun was gone they went out to work and play in the moonlight.

This went on for a very long time, and the family was very happy. However, there was one little boy in the family who was not happy. He yearned to be able to go outside in the daylight like all the other children. He yearned to feel the sun on his face, its warm rays on his skin.

One day the little boy opened the door. His sisters and brothers shouted, "Stop! You will be killed!" But no matter, the boy had to try. So he stepped out into the sun. He felt the wonderful touch of the rays on his face and on his skin. But it was so hot! It began to melt his eyes, his face, his arms, and his legs. Soon, he was nothing but a puddle of wax.

His wax brothers and sisters watched helplessly. They had to wait until the very last ray of light went behind the hills, before they could rush outside and stand around the puddle of him, weeping. Father scooped him up, shaped him into a little ball, and placed his remains in the branches of a tree. Then they all went home to mourn.

In the morning, everyone looked outside at the tree. But the ball of wax was gone. Instead, there was a beautiful bird of many striking colors, singing in the very place their brother had been left as a ball of wax. The bird looked at them, called out to them in song, then leapt into the air, spread its amazing wings against the sun, and flew away. From that day on, the bird returned every evening to sing its lovely song, and the family remembered their brother and son.

WORKING WITH THE STORY

ACTIVITIES

Contemplate this story during asana, meditation, or relaxation.

Make a list of things that must be destroyed to make something new: breaking eggs makes an omelet; grinding up beans makes coffee; food scraps become compost to fertilize new plants.

Look into a kaleidoscope. Notice the formation and reformation of shapes as you twist the cylinder. How does this happen? Do the old shapes die? Or do they change into something else?

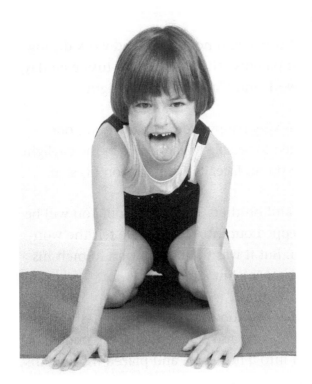

Talk about someone you know who has died. Remember that grief is a natural process, and it is okay to cry. What do you think happens when people die?

ASANA

A bird is a traditional symbol of the spirit and rebirth. After practicing asanas, realize that you are not the same person you were before starting the yoga practice. You are transformed and new again in the present moment. Roar like a **LION**, *simhasana*, and affirm this fact.

TREASURE: Peace

As part of a complex, diverse universe, we need an open mind that keeps us growing and learning. To be a voice for peace, we can first work on ourselves by practicing yoga and meditation and by guarding our actions, words, and deeds.

THE COLOR OF GOD – Africa

Out in the countryside of Africa lived two friends. One friend lived on the north side of the road, and the other friend lived on the south side of the road. Now one day, God decided to pay the friends a visit. He walked down the road when the two friends were outside in front tending their gardens. The right side of His face was painted red, while the left side of His face was painted blue. The two friends both stopped in awe and looked at God, who walked on by.

"Did you see God?" asked the friend on the north side of the street.

"Yes, I did! It was amazing!" said the friend on the south side of the street.

"Yes, his face was amazingly blue," said the friend on the north side of the street.

"Why, yes....no! Wait a minute! God wasn't blue! I saw Him myself, He was red!"

"What!" cried the friend from the north side. "No, no, no! You are absolutely wrong! He wasn't red at all! I saw Him! I know He was blue! I saw with my own eyes!"

"He was not!" cried the friend from the south side of the street, growing angry.

"He was blue!"

"He was red!"

The two friends started fighting and rolling in the dirt in the street. God decided to turn around and walk back down the street. This time the blue side of His face was shown to the friend on the south side and the red side of His face was shown to the friend on the north side. The two men stopped fighting, stood on their sides of the street, and once again watched in awe as God walked by.

"You were right!" cried the north friend. "He is red! I'm so sorry!"

"No, you were right. He is blue! I'm sorry!

"No, I said you were right and I'm wrong!" said the north friend, and he started to get angry again. Soon they were fighting and rolling in the dirt all over again.

WORKING WITH THE STORY

ACTIVITIES

Contemplate this story during asana, meditation, or relaxation.

Why do the friends continue to argue after they have solved their first disagreement? How can we get rid of our need to be right and make peace? Are you able to apologize when you have been wrong? How does it feel to apologize?

THE DOVE AND THE SPARROW – Unknown

A dove sat on a branch and watched a snowstorm. Later, a sparrow alighted next to the dove. The dove asked the sparrow, "Dear friend, tell me, what is the weight of a snowflake?"

The sparrow ruffled its feathers a bit and said, "Why, it's nothing. Absolutely nothing at all." The dove sat for a while contemplating this answer.

"Well, that is interesting," he said finally. "For I saw the most amazing thing. I was watching the snow fall, each tiny snowflake, one after another, as it gathered on a branch. More and more of these singular snowflakes gathered, until there was a great mound of snow on the branch. Still more snowflakes gathered, and then I saw the branch break. And you say that snowflakes weigh nothing."

The sparrow sat watching the snowfall without saying anything.

"I wonder," the dove said, "if that just like the snowflakes, all we need is one more voice, and we can finally have world peace."

WORKING WITH THE STORY

ACTIVITIES

Contemplate this story during asana practice, meditation, or relaxation.

How can we help others become peaceful? Can we teach others meditation, share our experience as an example of how to find peace? What can we do to help achieve world peace? Does one person make a difference?

ASANA

Find a tree, **TREE POSE**, *vrksasana*, and become a variety of birds. **EAGLE POSE**, *garudasana*. **CROW POSE**, *bakasana*. **PIGEON POSE**, *eka pada rajakapotanasana*. Come to rest in **SEATED FORWARD BEND**, *paschimotanasana*.

MEDITATION AND RELAXATION

Visualize a dove inside your heart. Hold that vision and fill the dove with love and dedication to work in service of world peace. Let the dove flutter away from the heart and into the sun, and know that this wish is granted.

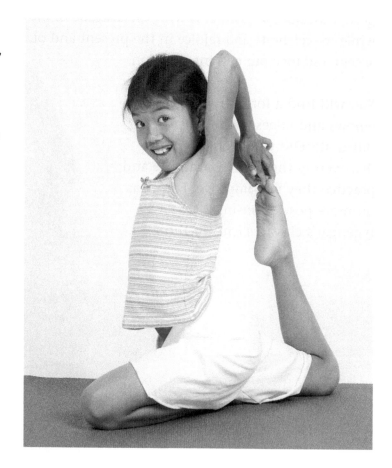

The Poses
Asanas

There are many yoga poses out there, more than I can possibly put in this little book. But here are many of the basic poses used in this book. Children will vary greatly in their flexibility and ability to perform the poses. Always see the beauty in the child's original pose and effort and honor that, while directing the child into the full alignment of the pose. Introduce adjustments with the attitude of moving toward something in process, while we celebrate and rejoice in the present and our practice of yoga and completely accept and love our current situation.

You will find a lot of hyper-extended elbows and knees, wobbly legs, etc. But that's OK! Guide children into discovering their bodies. In time and practice they will improve. For ideas on more poses, consult B.K.S. Iygengar's classic, *Light On Yoga*.

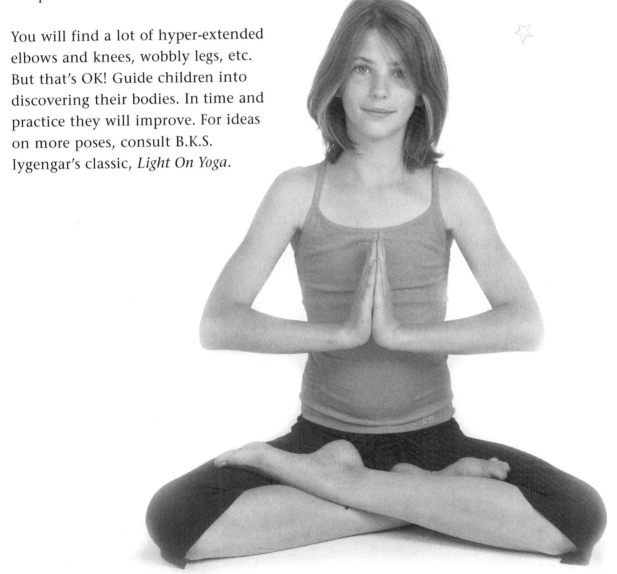

Basic Yoga Alignment
(based on Anusara yoga)

1. Open to grace. Breathing in and filling up with the beauty of ourselves, the gift and promise of now and our divine potential.

In standing position, the feet are fist width apart, with the second toe lined up with the middle of the ankle. Feet, ankles and legs are strong, drawing energy from the feet to the core of the pelvic area.

2. Muscular energy is achieved by drawing the muscles in toward each other.

3. Inner and 4. Outer Spiral is achieved by moving the inner thighs back, keeping them back, then tucking the tailbone.

5. Organic energy is achieved by extending out through the muscles and the bones, shining out the great, beautiful and powerful energy that we are into the world.

Shoulders should be on the back. Have children shrug their shoulders by their ears, then take the shoulders back. There should not be a "banana back" with the low back way in. The tailbone should be tucked and the kidney area should be full.

In bent knee poses, such as lunges, knees should be over the ankles.

When in table position, children's fingers should be spread wide, like the rays of the sun, and wrist joints straight across. All fingers should be strongly on the floor.

ALIGNMENT CHECK!

Periodically throughout class, I have an alignment check. Starting with the toes if children are in standing position. Call out, "Feet check!" and check children's alignment of their feet. Demonstrate what out of alignment is, such as toes pointing outwards like a duck, too far in like a pigeon. Help children correct their alignment.

Do the same thing with, "Hand check," keeping fingers spread wide, "Knee check!" ensuring that children's knees are over their ankles, "Shoulder check" such as in cobra pose, *bhujangasana*, that shoulders are on the back instead of sloped forward.

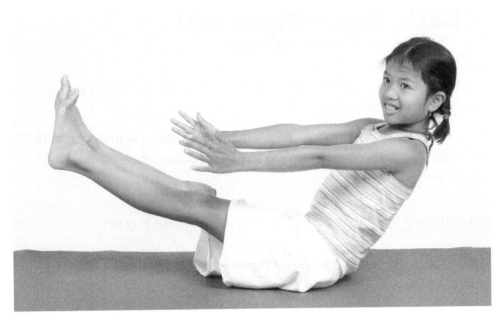

BOAT POSE

Navasana

Begin seated with knees bent. Bring arms
out straight in front near knees. Use stomach
muscles to draw legs in and up. Extend legs
out for full position.

HALF BOAT POSE

Ardha Navasana

From boat pose, lower the body
half way down and use stomach
muscles to hover.

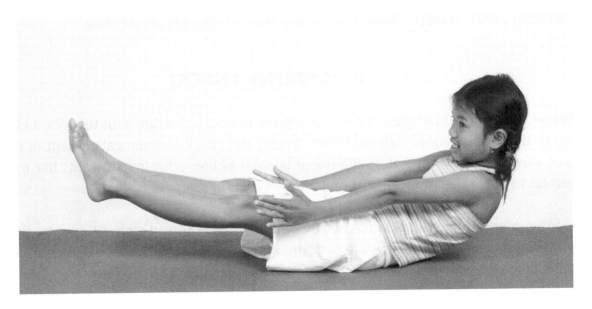

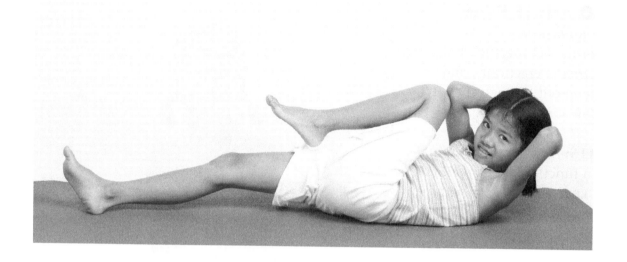

KNEE TO ELBOW POSE

Lace fingers behind the head. Draw left knee to chest and right elbow to left knee. Switch to drawing right knee in and left elbow to knee. Switch back and forth quickly.

BENEFITS: Strengthens abdominals, improves digestion. Tones the kidneys.

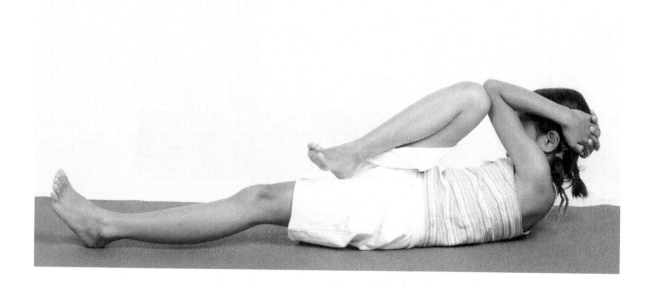

BOUND ANGLE POSE

Baddha Konasana

Seated, bring feet together. Press feet together energetically, and then extend out through the knees. Bow forward.

BENEFITS: Aids lower abdominal organs in functioning. Good for hip and knee joints. Helps with bladder control.

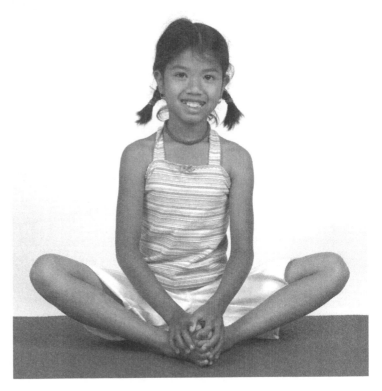

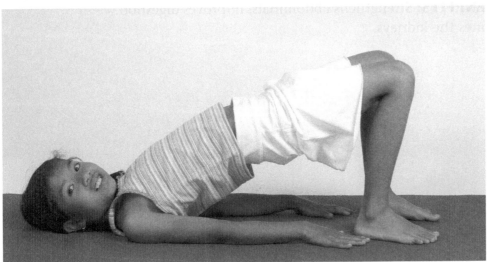

BRIDGE POSE

Setu Bandha Sharvangasana

Begin lying on back. Bend knees and bring feet toward buttocks. Press hips up. Walk shoulder blades underneath and then clasp hands. Keep inner thighs moving toward each other and tuck the tailbone.

BENEFITS: Opens the chest and upper back. Develops the buttocks.

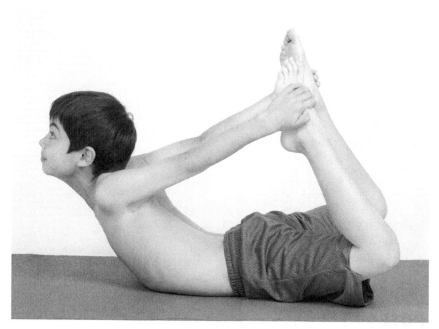

BOW POSE
Dhanurasana
Begin lying face down. Bend knees. Bring shoulders on the back and grab ankles. Tuck the tailbone and arch up. Rock side to side for variation.

BENEFITS: Stretches the spine and keeps it flexible. Tones the abdominal organs.

CAMEL POSE
Ustrasana
Kneeling with toes curved under or flat on the floor, place hands on hips. Extend and lift the spine as you arch the back. Drop the hands back onto the heels, press the hips forward, tuck tailbone.

BENEFITS: Develops hamstrings and inner thighs. Calms the mind and removes fatigue. Removes stiffness in the neck and shoulders.

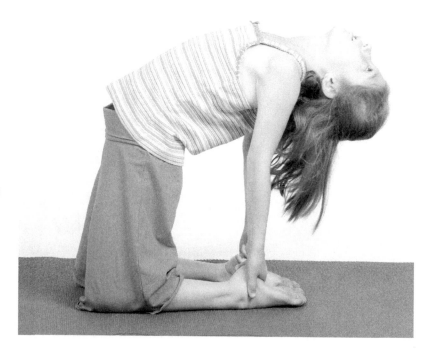

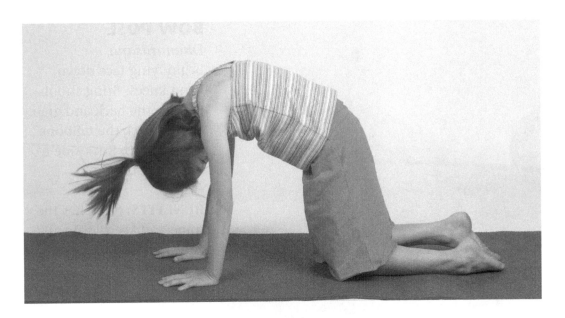

CAT/COW POSE
Bidalasana

Beginning in table pose, inhale. Exhale and arch back up like a cat.
Inhale again and drop down like a cow.

BENEFITS: Good for the spine. Develops the wrists and arms.

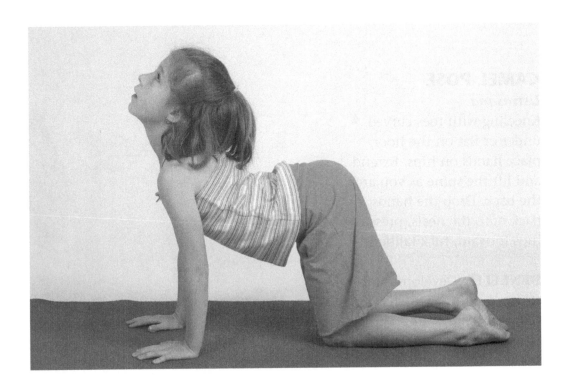

CHAIR POSE

Utkatasana

Begin in mountain pose. Raise arms over head, bend knees and bring together and sit as if sitting in a chair.

BENEFITS: Strengthens ankles, calves, inner thighs, back. Stretches the shoulders.

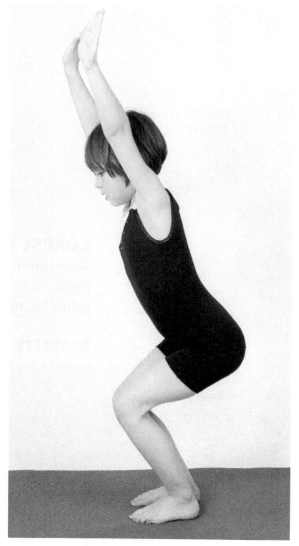

CHILD'S POSE

Balasana

Have child spread knees and extend arms forward in front of them. Also may move arms to the sides.

BENEFITS: A good resting pose. Good for the back.

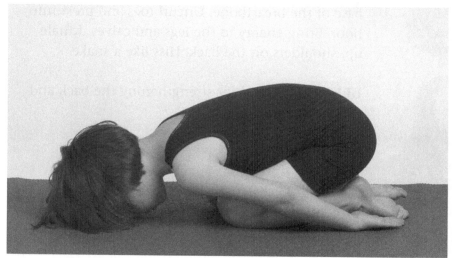

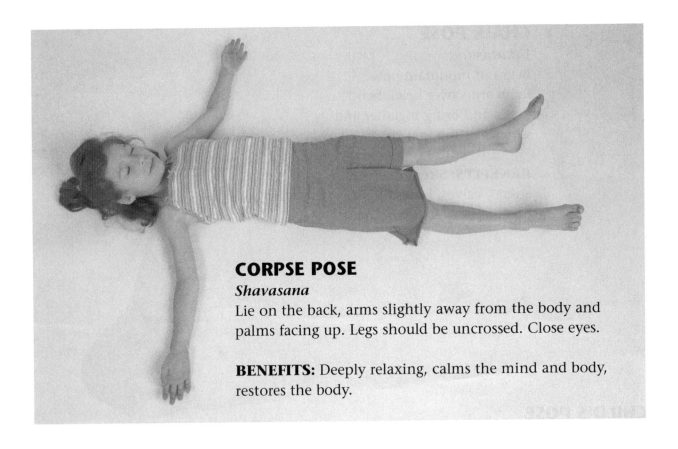

CORPSE POSE
Shavasana
Lie on the back, arms slightly away from the body and palms facing up. Legs should be uncrossed. Close eyes.

BENEFITS: Deeply relaxing, calms the mind and body, restores the body.

COBRA POSE
Bhujangasana
Begin lying flat on stomach, hands back by the base of the breastbone. Uncurl toes and press into floor. Bring energy to the legs and calves. Inhale up, shoulders on the back. Hiss like a snake.

BENEFITS: Good for strengthening the back and spine. Expands the chest.

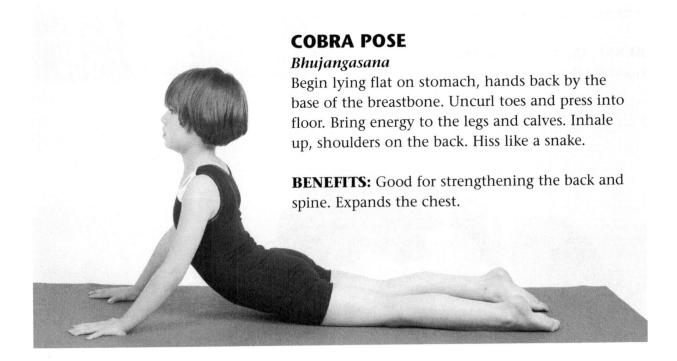

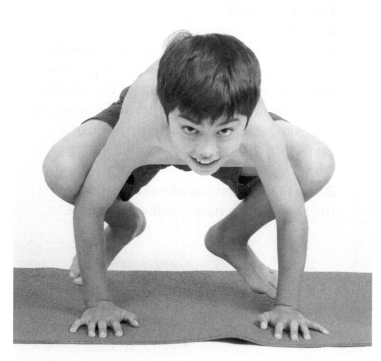

CROW POSE
Bakasana
Squat with feet together and place hands palm face down on floor with elbows bent. Rest knees onto backs of upper arms. Take away one foot and balance on one foot at first, then drawing into the core, balance and pull other foot up as well.

BENEFITS: Strengthens the arms and abdominal organs.

DOWNWARD DOG POSE
Adho Mukha Svanasana
Begin in table pose. Lean back toward heels, then press hips and buttocks up and back. Straighten legs.

BENEFITS: Removes fatigue, develops the ankles, arms and abdominals, strengthens and relieves stiffness in shoulders, good for digestion.

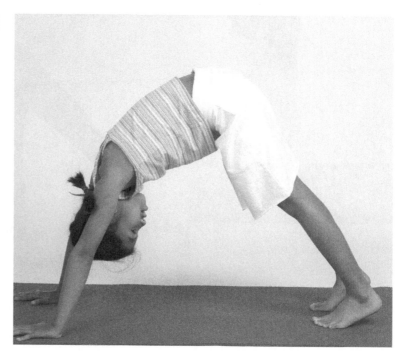

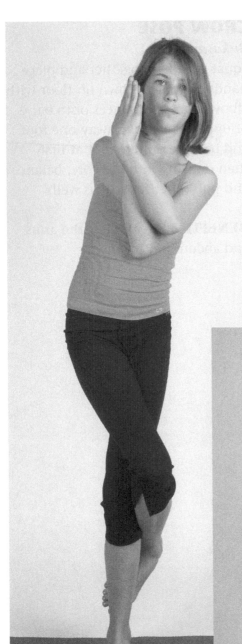

EAGLE POSE

Garudasana

Begin standing in mountain pose. Entwine left leg over the right leg. Extend right arm out, then cross left over it. Bend the elbows and entwine the two together and bring hands together. Release and fly out like an eagle. Switch sides.

BENEFITS: Strengthens ankles, stretches the shoulders, removes cramps in calves.

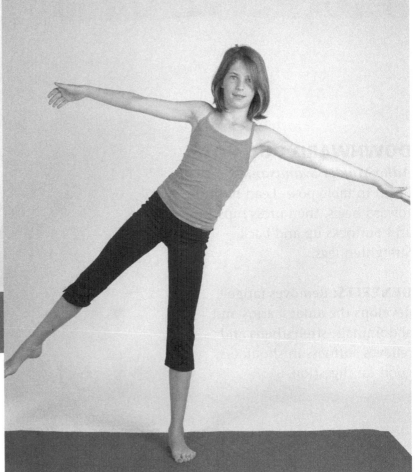

FEATHER DANCER POSE

Natarajasana

Begin standing on one leg and
bring knee to hands. Bring right
hand to hold right big toe. Then
arch back and tuck tailbone. Press
foot into hand. Extend left hand
out and bow forward. Balance.
Reverse sides.

BENEFITS: Strengthens leg
muscles, develops poise.
Stretches the shoulder blade
area and expands the chest.
Benefits the spine.

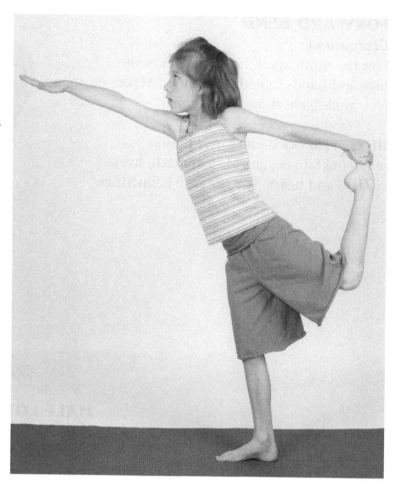

FISH POSE

Matsyasana

Sit on hands, palms facing down. Legs are extended. Drop elbows down to floor and
arch back. Slide back enough so that head will touch the floor.

BENEFITS: Good for the abdominal organs.

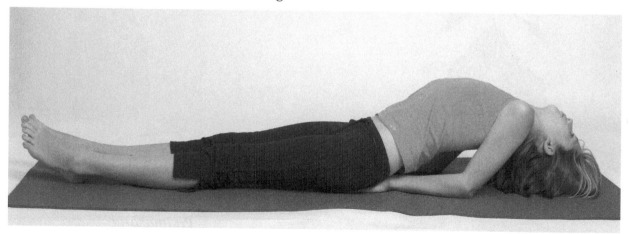

FORWARD BEND

Uttanasana

Feet fist width apart, bending over at the hips and hands touching the floor. Make feet, ankles, knees and legs strong.

BENEFITS: Good for concentration, removing fatigue, good for stomach, liver, kidneys and heart. Stretches the hamstrings.

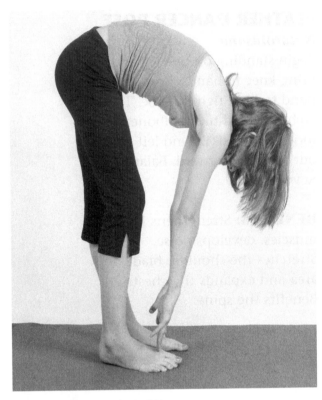

HALF LOTUS POSE

Ardha Padmasana

Seated, as in criss-cross apple sauce. Some children may be able to do the full lotus.

BENEFITS: Helps with relaxation and calms the mind.

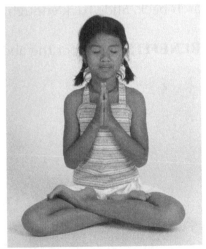

FULL LOTUS POSE

Padmasana

HALF MOON POSE
Ardha Chandrasana

From triangle pose, bend right knee and take a small step with left foot. Balance on right foot, extend left leg out. Right hand is on the floor, left hand extends out. Try looking at fingertips.

BENEFITS: Good for legs and lower spine. Strengthens knees. Good for balance.

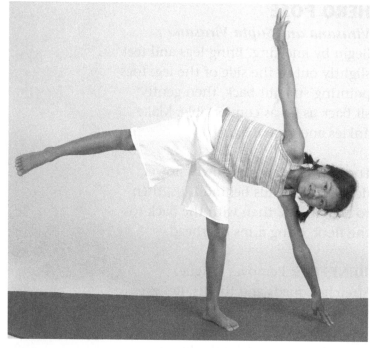

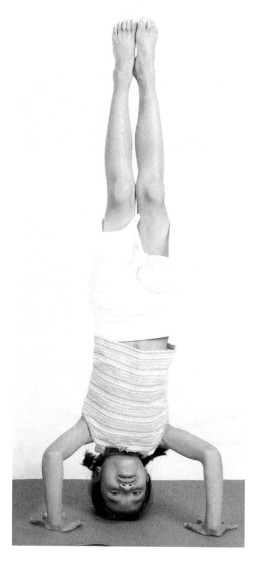

HEADSTAND
Sirsasana II

Every child I know loves headstand. Kids are naturals at it. It's considered the king of poses, or one of the most important because of its benefits. I do stress the importance of supervision and safety in this pose, however.

Place palms parallel to each other and fingers pointing toward the head shoulder width apart. Bring knees toward the head and place the crown of the head on the floor. Raise the knees from the floor and stretch the legs straight. Keep thighs energized and moving toward each other. Extend legs and feet into the air.

BENEFITS: Balance and poise. Energizes the body. Gives a healthy flow of blood through the brain cells, rejuvenation of brain cells.

HERO POSE

Virasana and Supta Virasana

Begin by kneeling. Bring legs and feet slightly out to the side of the leg, toes pointing straight back, then gently sit back as far as comfortable. Make ankles and toes active.

For reclined version, slowly slower down with hands behind hips, then to the elbows, then with the back to the floor, bring arms overhead.

BENEFITS: Removes fatigue. Stretches quads and thighs. Relieves stomach problems. Calms the mind. Encourages deep breathing and a rested heart. Good for the knees. Opens the chest.

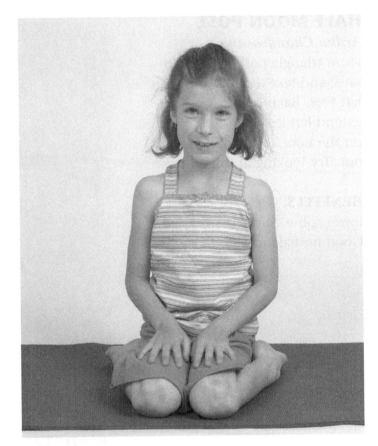

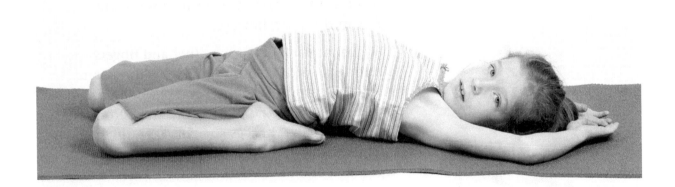

LION POSE
Simhasana

Start in child's pose with arms and hands extended. Then press forward and let face go wild. Squish it up! Roar like a lion!

BENEFITS: Good for the speech and stammers. Releases tension in the face and body and revives expression!

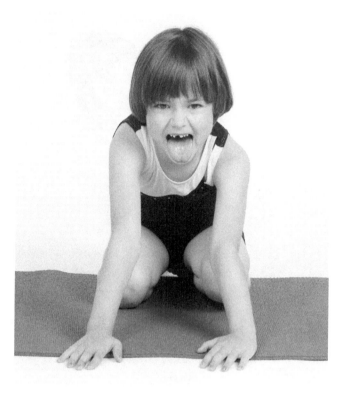

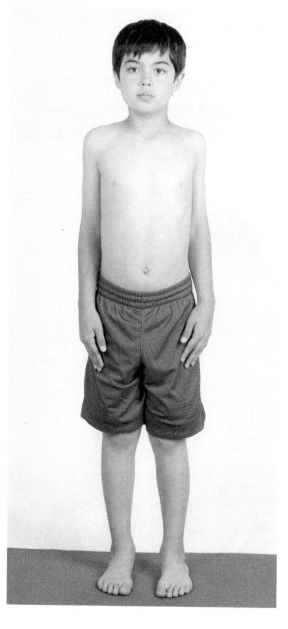

MOUNTAIN POSE
Tadasana

Stand with feet fist width apart. Weight evenly distributed through all four corners of the feet. Muscles of the ankles, calves, knees and thighs engaged and hugging the bones. Shoulders are on the back, hands pointed down. Feel the energy from the earth and feet drawing up into the core and extending out through the hands and head and feet.

BENEFITS: Teaches to stand properly. Develops concentration. Makes back strong.

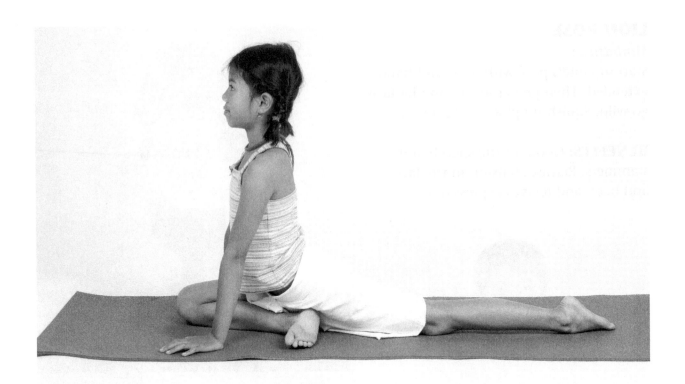

PIGEON POSE

Eka Pada Rajakapotasana

Begin in table position. Bring one knee forward and rotate leg open a bit. Extend back leg out. Bow forward. Switch sides. Try full pigeon and bend back leg, extend arm up and over to grab back toe. Lift up and tuck the tailbone to get there!

BENEFITS: Opens the hips, stretches the legs.

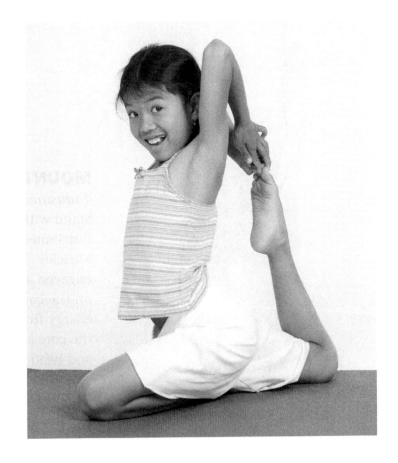

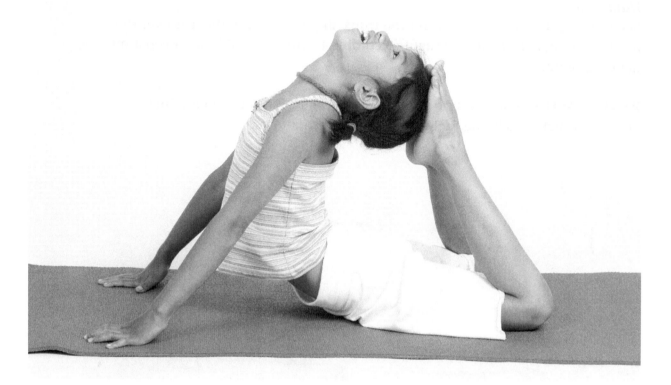

PRETTY POSE

Rajakapotasana

For the advanced pose, bend the knees and lift the feet up. Stretch spine and neck until head rests on the heels.

PLOW POSE

Halasana

Begin in shoulderstand, then lower the trunk slightly to bring the legs over the head. Knees may be bent or straight, according to children's abilities. Keep arms flat on ground,

BENEFITS: Has same effects as shoulderstand, rejuvenates the abdominal organs and helps backache. Helps stiff arms and shoulders.

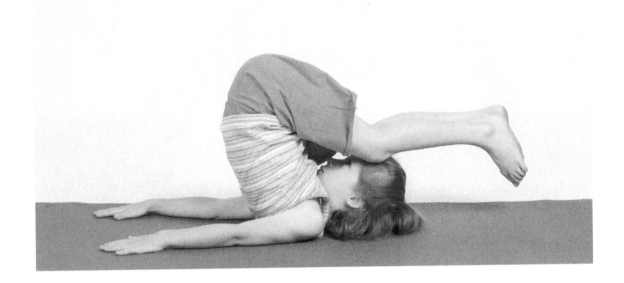

RABBIT POSE

Sasangasana

Begin in table position. Place hands on ankles, then arch the back and tuck head under. Place gentle weight on head.

BENEFITS: Stretches the back, arms and neck.

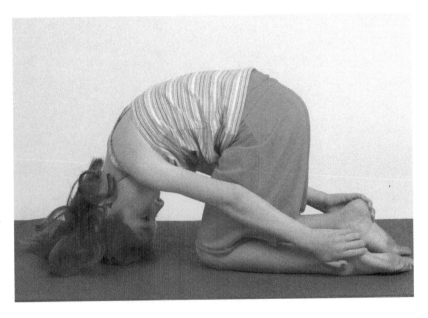

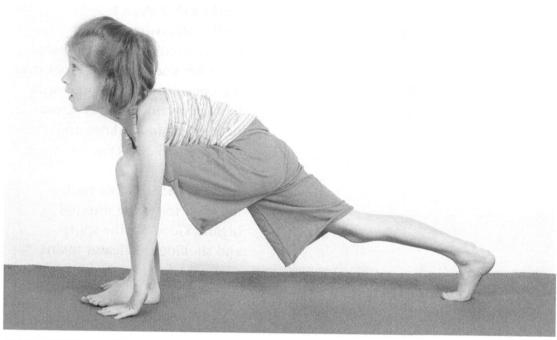

RUNNER'S LUNGE

Begin in downward dog. Lunge right foot forward with knee at right angle above the ankle. Bring shoulders on the back and extend out through back heel.

BENEFITS: Stretches the legs and psoas muscle.

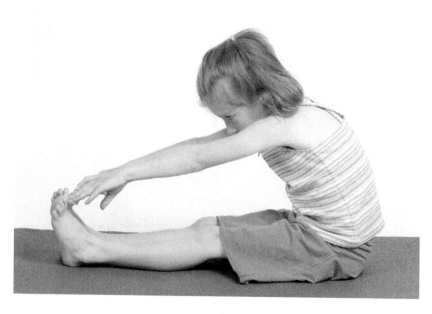

SEATED FORWARD BEND

Paschimotanasana
Sit on floor with legs extended. Bow forward and touch toes.

BENEFITS: Tones the abdominal organs, kidneys and is good for the spine.

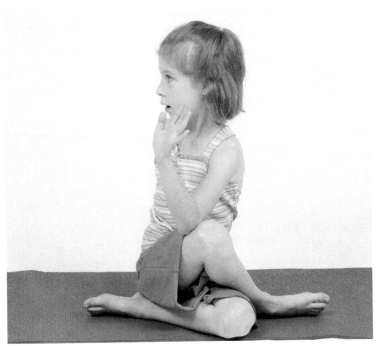

SEATED TWIST
Ardha Matsydendrasana
Begin seated with legs extended. Bend left knee and place foot over the opposite leg. Bring opposite foot in toward buttocks. Cross right elbow to left knee and leverage back. Reverse.

BENEFITS: Stretches neck muscles. Tones the internal organs. Good for the spine and shoulders. Releases toxins.

SHOULDERSTAND
Salamba Sharvangasana
Begin lying on the floor, then bend the knees. Keep hands and arms on the floor, palms down. Draw the legs in toward the stomach, then raise hips from the floor. Raise the trunk up supported by the hands until the chest touches the chin.

BENEFITS: Called the "mother of asanas" by Iyengar, has many uses, including thyroid, restoration of the body, circulation and sinus problems.

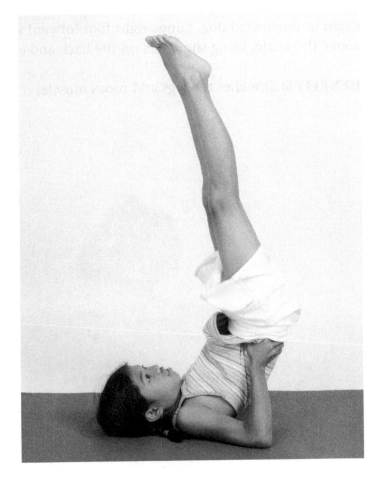

TRIANGLE POSE

Trikonasana

Spread legs wide on the mat, left foot turned in at 90 degrees and right foot pointing straight out. Inhale arms up to shoulder height. Bring muscular energy to the legs and arms, then extend trunk over to the right leg and bring the right hand toward the right ankle. Left arm extends straight up. Look at the fingertips. Switch sides.

BENEFITS: Strengthens leg muscles and ankles, builds the chest.

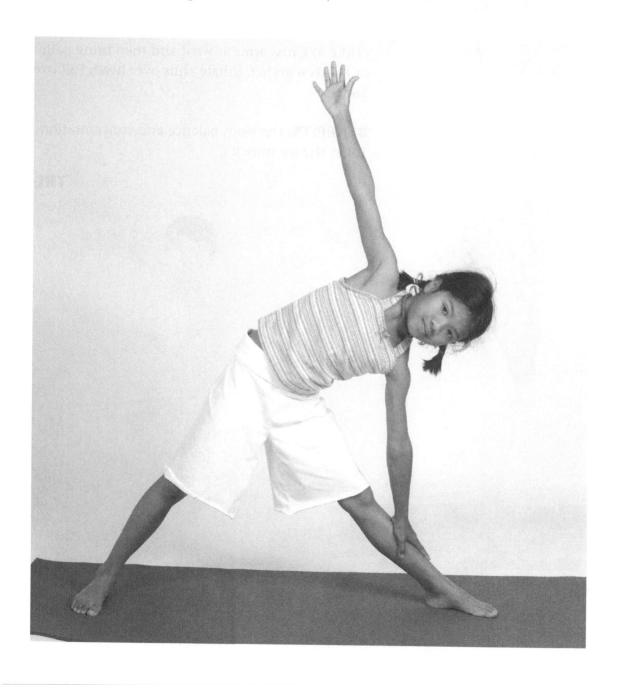

TREE POSE

Vrksasana

Begin in mountain pose. Put weight onto right leg and then lift left foot to the right thigh, toes pointing downwards. Balancing, lift arms up overhead, palms together. (TREE 1) Flower the tree (TREE 2) by opening the hands and bringing arms down to the sides again. Switch sides.

Twisty branches (TREE 3) waving in the wind. (TREE 4) Cross arms at wrist and then bring palms of hands together. Inhale arms over head. Fall over. Timber!

BENEFITS: Develops balance and concentration. Tones the leg muscles.

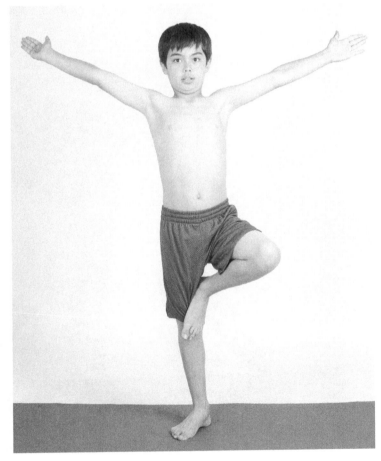

TREE 2

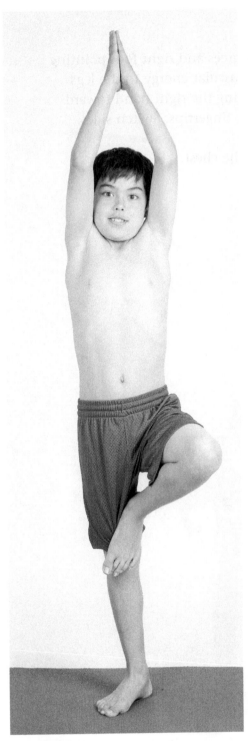

TREE 1

TREE 3

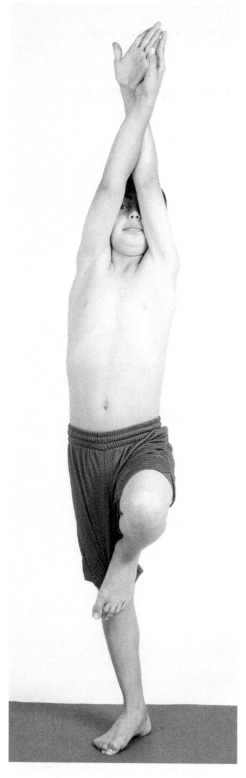

TREE 4

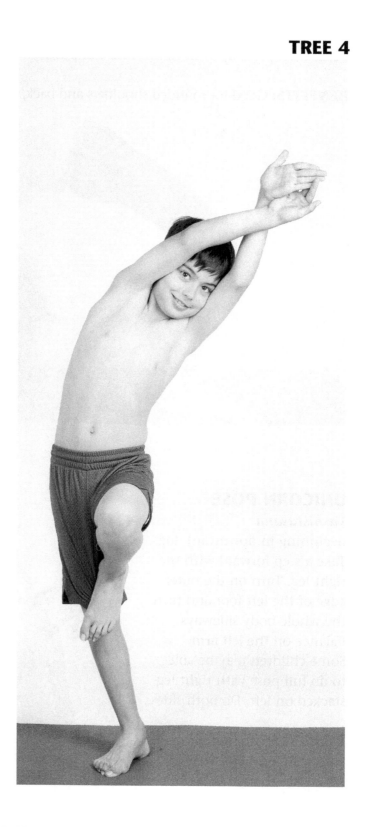

UPWARD FACING BOW POSE

Urdva Dhanurasana

Place hands behind shoulders before pressing up into bridge pose. Come up onto head, then press up with hands into full pose.

BENEFITS: Good for rounded shoulders and back, aids respiration, improves energy.

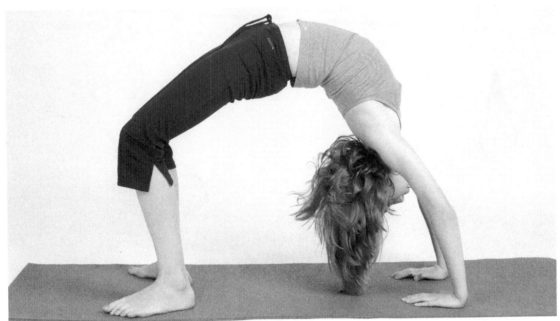

UNICORN POSE

Vashistasana

Beginning in downward dog. Take a step forward with the right leg. Turn on the outer edge of the left foot and turn the whole body sideways. Balance on the left arm. Some children may be able to do full pose with right leg stacked on left. Do both sides.

BENEFITS: Strengthens the wrists, strengthens the legs and tones the spine.

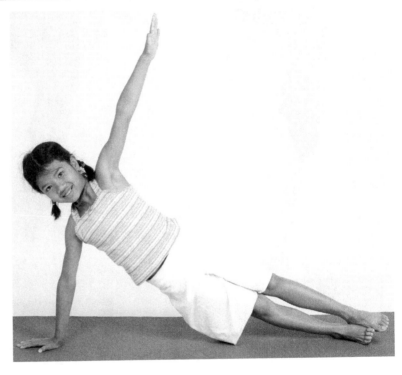

WARRIOR I

Virabhadrasana I

Spread legs wide. Turn left foot in and right foot out. Bend left knee to a 90-degree angle, extend arms up overhead. Do both sides.

BENEFITS: Opens up shoulders, back and the neck and strengthens them. Develops good breathing in the chest. Builds stamina, strengthens legs, ankles and knees.

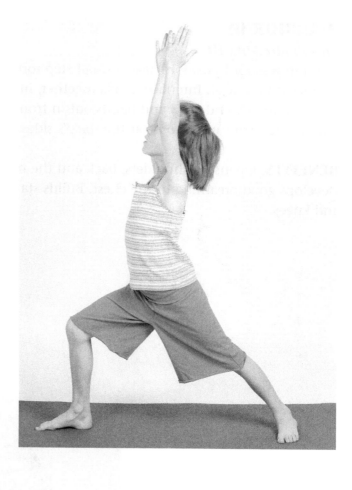

WARRIOR II

Virabhadrasana II

Spread legs wide. Turn left foot in and right foot out. Bend left knee to a 45-degree angle, extend right arms out in front and left arm behind. Do both sides.

BENEFITS: Opens up shoulders, back and the neck and strengthens them. Develops good breathing in the chest. Builds stamina, strengthens legs, ankles and knees.

WARRIOR III

Virabhadrasana III

Begin in warrior I position. Take a small step forward with back right foot. Balance on left foot. Interlace hands together, index fingers and thumbs together and extend arms and hands out in front. Extend right leg straight out behind. Arms can also be at the torso's sides. Do both sides.

BENEFITS: Opens up shoulders, back and the neck and strengthens them. Develops good breathing in the chest. Builds stamina. Strengthens legs, ankles and knees.

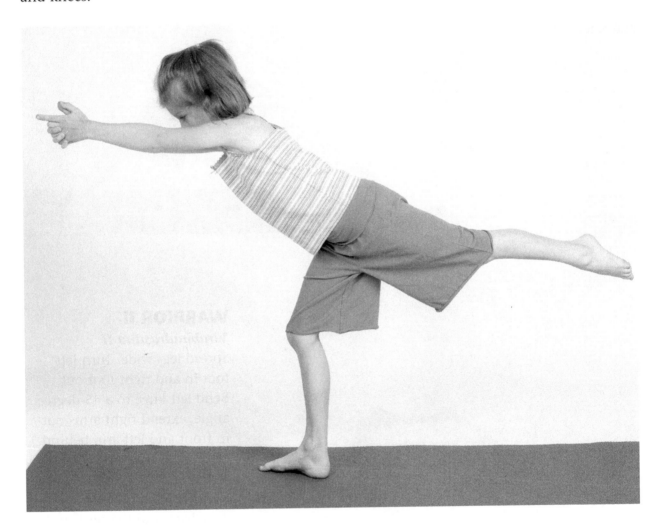

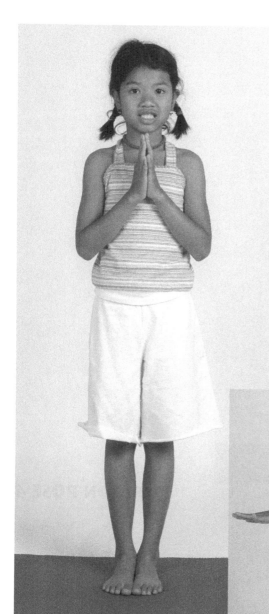

MOON SALUTATION
Vinyasa

(MOON 1) Mountain pose
(MOON 2) Jump legs apart
(MOON 3) Triangle
(MOON 4) Runner's lunge
(MOON 5) Half moon
(MOON 6) Standing splits
(MOON 7) Warrior II

(MOON 2) Return to legs apart
(MOON 1) Back to mountain pose

MOON POSE 2

MOON POSE 1

MOON POSE 3

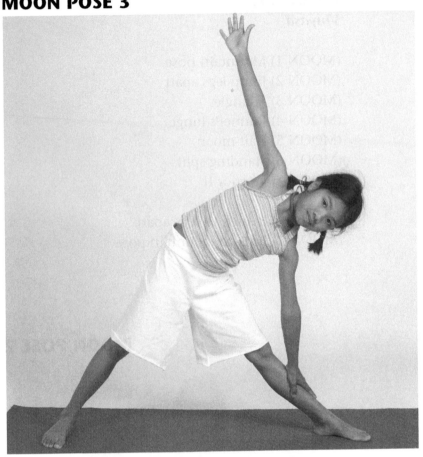

MOON POSE 4

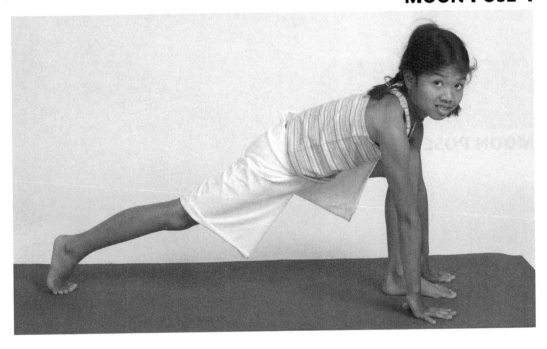

MOON POSE 5

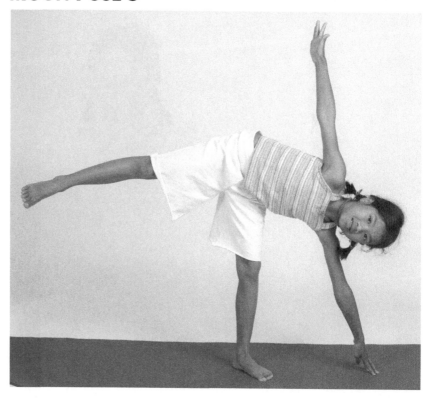

MOON POSE 6

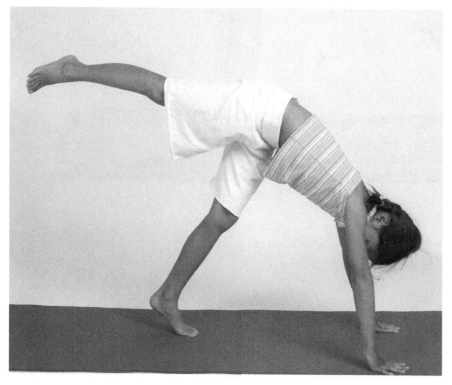

MOON POSE 7

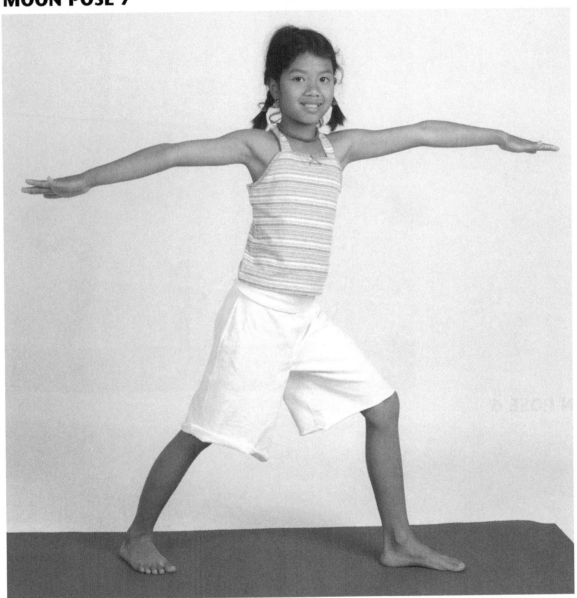

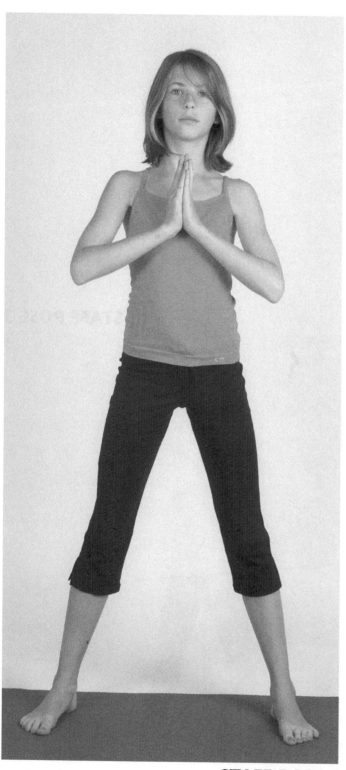

STAFF POSE 1

STAFF OF BRAHMA
Vinyasa

(STAFF 1) begin with legs spread apart, hands in prayer position and inhale

(STAFF 2) exhale and dive forward with the hands and arms outstretched in front

(STAFF 3) inhale and part the arms to the side

(STAFF 4) exhale turn palms face up

(STAFF 5) inhale arms up over head

(STAFF 6) exhale and looking at the floor bow forward

(STAFF 7) inhale and look forward, reaching, reaching

(STAFF 8) then exhale and drop to the floor, knees slightly bent

(STAFF 9) inhale roll up the spine

(STAFF 10) exhale at the hips

(STAFF 11) and then inhale arms up over head again

(STAFF 12) exhale hands back into prayer position and bend knees

Repeat 3 times

STAFF POSE 2

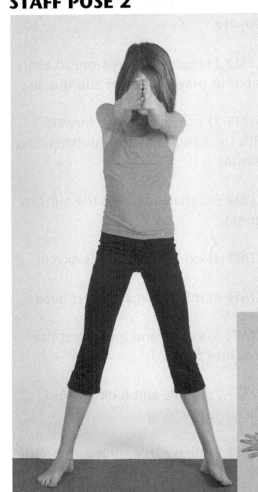

STAFF POSE 3

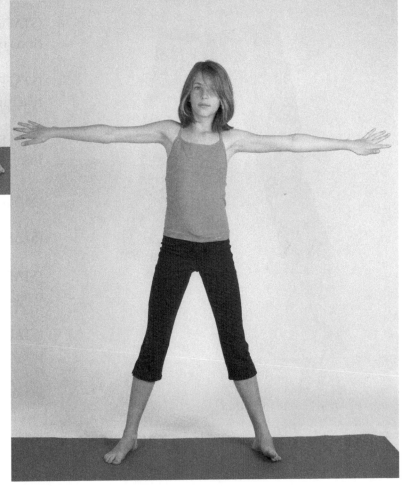

STAFF POSE 4

STAFF POSE 5

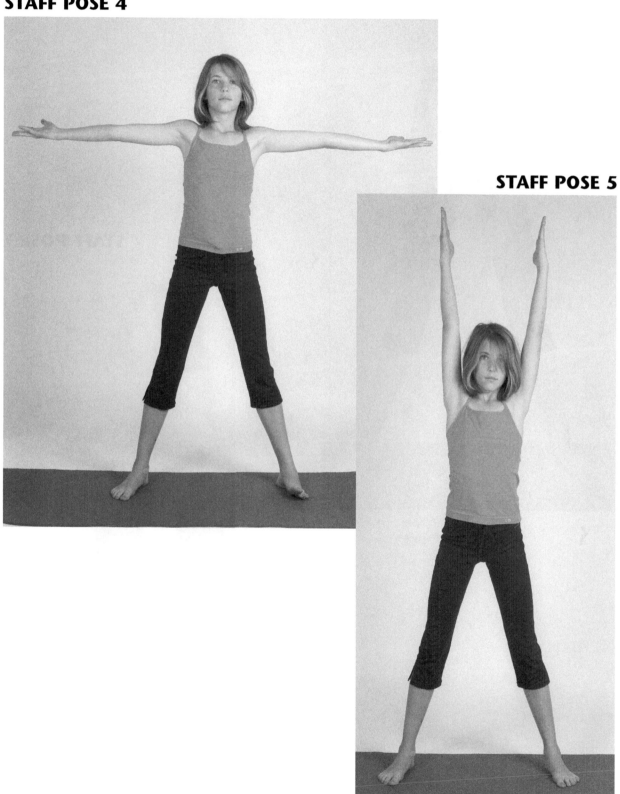

STAFF POSE 6

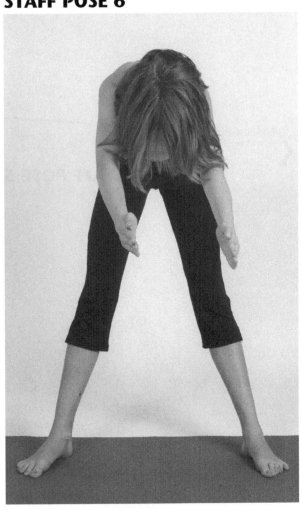

STAFF POSE 7

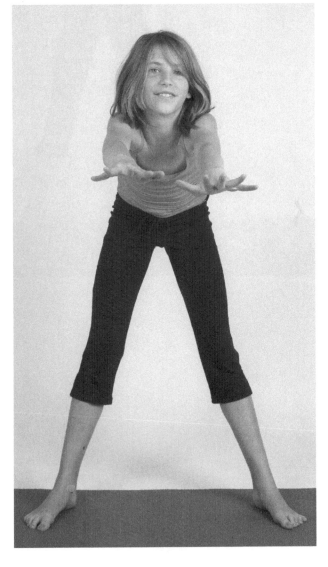

STAFF POSE 8

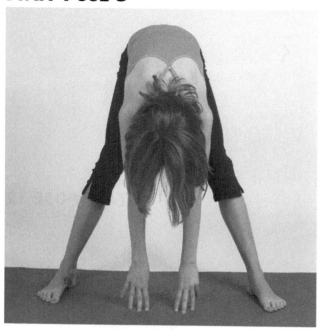

STAFF POSE 9

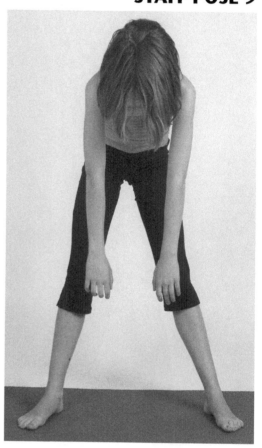

STAFF POSE 10

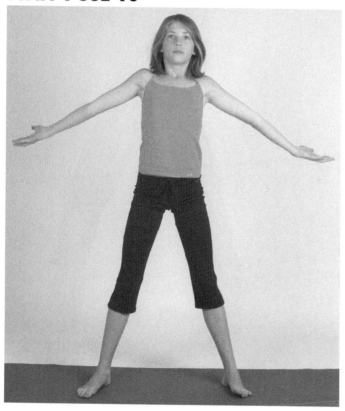

STAFF POSE 11

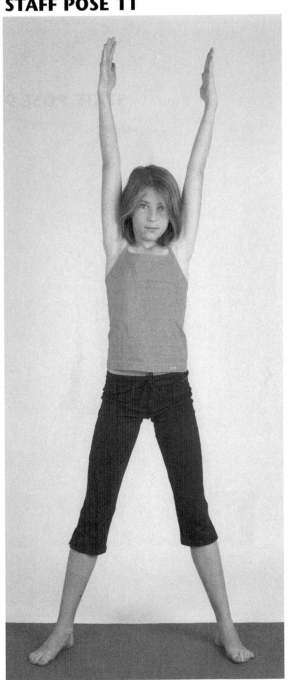

STAFF POSE 12

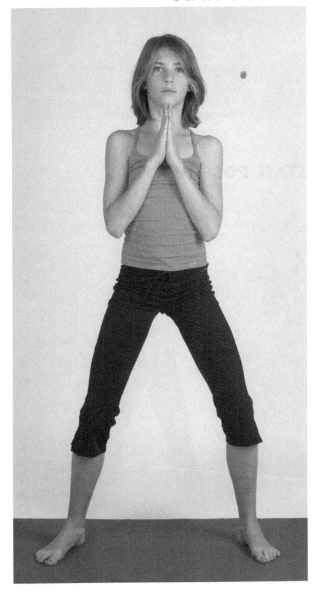

Appendix:

Using Interfaith Stories and
Teaching Yoga in the Public Schools

Mythologist Joseph Campbell said that one person's religion is another person's mythology. We may be offended to consider our religion a "myth," but myth comes from the Greek word *mythos*, which means story. According to Campbell, the human mind cannot access the ineffable transcendence of God without myth and story. The word religion comes from the Latin *religio* – to re-link, and it is through storytelling that we link ourselves to the divine within ourselves.

In his book, *The Hero with a Thousand Faces*, Campbell tells us that all the world's religions and cultures have a common hero theme. Humans have always been on a quest for the divine, and in fact the divine is found within us, in our unity with the entire universe. Mythology provides the road map to find this reunion.

> …we have not even to risk the adventure alone; for the heroes of all time have gone before us; the labyrinth is thoroughly known; we have only to follow the thread of the hero-path. And where we had thought to find an abomination, we shall find a god; where we had thought to slay another, we shall slay ourselves; where we had thought to travel outward, we shall come to the center of our own existence; where we had thought to be alone, we shall be with all the world.

Because we can present yoga from an interfaith and mythological standpoint, it is well suited for public schools. When I teach yoga, I do not proselytize; I do not even teach "spirituality." I teach self-esteem and mental health with yoga, and I find that the interfaith stories presented in this book serve that purpose, and teach yoga universally. How do the children react? In one after-school program I taught, a little girl always said that she saw Jesus in her heart during *shavasana*. Another girl was an atheist and said, "I don't believe that. I saw something else." I honored each child's ability to say what they believed and felt. My class provided the space for acknowledgement and acceptance of each student's individual search for happiness and meaning. The stories in this book speak to Hindus, Muslims, Christians, Jews, Wiccans, atheists, and others. Yoga is what you bring to it.

To find peace, we must be aware that the truth is unlimited; there is no untruth in another religion's teaching. In *The Sermon on the Mount According to Vedanta*, Swami Prabhavandanda says that Christianity cannot be the sole originator of the truth of God. It would not be truth; for truth cannot be originated; it exists. He recounts St. Augustine as saying,

> That which is called the Christian religion existed among the ancients,
> and never did not exist from the beginning of the human race until
> Christ came in the flesh, at which time the true religion, which
> already existed, began to be called Christianity.

In my classes, I say sometimes we are going to hear a story about Jesus, and sometimes we are going to hear a story about the Buddha or Allah or the Great Spirit or nothing at all. I teach that this expands our minds, expands our possibilities, and makes us unlimited.

I teach my students that we show respect when we listen to each other's stories. By allowing ourselves to witness different perspectives, we sacrifice our need to be right. We can still believe in our stories and let others believe in theirs, too. We can see the commonality in the stories, and we can see that indeed all of these stories have the same themes: the search for happiness, the search for God and wholeness, the joys, pains, sorrows, and fears of life. When we listen to each other's stories, we realize that there is only one story in the world — the human story.

When we start to examine our own stories using the *yamas* and the *niyamas* of Patanjali's 8-fold path, we realize that we have been mis-identifying with the mind and the mind's story. Something happens to us in our life, and we make it mean something. We carry this story around – which exists only in memory, *smriti* – and we begin to identify with it. It takes us out of the present and allows us to be consumed with the fear and desire of I, me, and mine. We lose sight of our connection to the divine.

Yoga stories free us to look beyond the barriers of gender, socio-economic situation, and race. When we can relate our lives to these larger stories, we make connections to a larger meaning. Then we encounter those ah-ha moments that ultimately bring peace.

As we go deeper in the practice of yoga, we find that we are not separate from one another. In Hinduism, it is said that the universe is threaded together by Indra's net — where the net is stranded together by jewels, and each jewel is reflecting the others, and each jewel sees itself in the other jewel. We need each other to see ourselves, to make sense of the world, to find community and love. Otherwise, like Jonah in the belly of the whale, the loneliness of facing our inner selves is unbearable. Man is not meant to be separate from the divine, from his fellows, or from himself.

Occasionally, parents of public school children who may not be familiar with yoga may feel threatened by the practice. Some fundamentalists fear that by going inward, their children may encounter "the devil." I try to reassure these parents that the guilt and fear produced by separation from Self is itself a form of evil, but often I find it easiest to refer to yoga as movement and meditation as silence. We should always remind the adults that these are tools for discipline and character education. The positive result of the children's yoga practice — the improvement in school performance, the benefits to mental health, and the overall sense of calm the children exude — will become the best advocates for the course.

Story Sources

All of these stories are traditional folk tales. I have heard them numerous times throughout my life. Some may have appeared in other sources than the ones listed below.

THE JEWEL IN THE WELL
I came upon this story during my experience as a Spellbinders storyteller. See www.Spellbinder.org. I have not found a written source; however, the motif appears elsewhere. In Rafe Martin's book, *One Hand Clapping: Zen Stories for All Ages*, (Rizzoli Publications, New York, 1995), a Zen monk is awarded a small silver statue of a cat that is worth a great deal. When the monk sees some children playing with clay animals, he gives it to them without another thought and walks away.

THE ROAR OF AWAKENING
I found this story in several places: *Folktales from India*, by A.K. Ramanujan (Pantheon Books, New York, 1991), *Philosophies of India*, by Heinric Zimmer (Princeton University Press, 1951), *The Gospel of Sri Ramakrishna*, translated with an introduction by Swami Nikhilananda (New York, 1942), and in Healing Story Alliance list serve, www.HealingStory.org.

BRAHMA'S TEARS
I heard this story from storyteller Angela Lloyd, who got it from the Healing Through Story list serve, www.HealingStory.org. Another variant comes from the Sufi poet Hafiz, in the book *The Gift, Poems by Hafiz*, translated by Daniel Ladinsky (Penguin Compass, New York, 1999). Another version can be found in *Soul Food, Stories to Nourish the Spirit and the Heart* by Jack Kornfield and Christina Feldman (Harper, San Francisco, 1991).

THE CRACKED POT
I first heard this story from my sister, Narada Dasi Johnson, and also my yoga teacher, Bhakti. Some call it a Hindu story, and some call it a Christian story, but I have not found a written source.

THE MONKEY AND THE MOON

I first heard this story from Tai Chi master Chuangliang Al Huang at the Esalen Institute. There is a Sufi version with Nassrudin in *The Moon in the Well: Wisdom Tales to Transform Your Life, Family, and Community* by Erica Helm Mead, (Open Court, Pap/Com edition, 2001). A Persian version can be found in, *Parabola*, (Winter 2003, vol. 28, no. 4). There is a Tibetan version in Margaret Read McDonalds' *Peace Tales: World Folktale to Talk About*, (August House, Little Rock, 2005). Many will be familiar with the Aesop story of the dog with the bone that sees his reflection in the water, thinks it's another dog, plunges in to fight the dog, and loses his bone.

THE STONECUTTER

I first heard this story as a Spellbinder storyteller. There is also a written version beautifully done by Caldecott-winning author and friend Gerald McDermott. (Viking Press, New York, 1975)

GIFT FROM THE GODS

I heard this from the Healing Story Alliance list serve, www.HealingStory.org. Some believe that the tale comes from India, but I could not track it down.

THE STORY OF THE SANDS

This story is found in *Tales of the Dervishes*, by Idries Shah (Plume, 1970). *The Tree of Yoga* by BKS Iyengar (Shambhala Publications, Boston, 1988), makes reference to this motif.

THE THREE SISTERS

This story comes from *Indonesian Legends and Folk Tales*, by Adele De Leeuw (Thomas Nelson & Sons, New York, 1964).

CALMING THE STORM

Sources for this story include: *The Aquarian Gospel of Jesus the Christ*, Levi, DeVorss & Co. (Santa Monica, California, 1907), *The Children's Bible*, (Golden Press, New York), and *The Thompson Chain-Reference Bible* (B.B. Kirkbride Bible Co. Inc. Indianapolis, Indiana, 1988).

THE BANYAN DEER

I found this story in several places, including *Buddhist Birth Stories or Jataka Tales*, by Rhys Davids (Arno Press, New York, 1977).

MOHAMMAD AND THE CAT

Mohammad was said to have been very kind to animals. According to a report (*hadith*) attributed to Abu Huraira, he owned a cat named Muezza, about whom it is said that one day while she was asleep on the sleeve of Mohammad's robe, the call to prayer was sounded. Rather than awaken the cat, Mohammad quietly cut his sleeve off and left. When he returned, the cat bowed to him and thanked him, after which she was guaranteed a place in heaven. This story is also found in Elisa Davy Pearmain's *Doorways to the Soul, 52 Wisdom Tales From Around the World* (The Pilgrim Press, Cleveland, Ohio, 1998).

PRAYING THE PSALMS

I found this story in *The Soul's Almanac, a Year of Interfaith Stories, Prayers and Wisdom* by Aaron Zerah (Putnam, New York, 1998). This is also known as the folk tale, *The Three Sillies*, and I thank Elisa Pearmain for bringing it to my attention. A version can be found in *The Children's Hour, Favorite Fairy Tales*, by Marjorie Barrows (Grolier Inc., New York, 1966).

WALKING ON WATER

This story is also in *The Soul's Almanac, a Year of Interfaith Stories, Prayers and Wisdom*. A Tibetan version can be found in Parabola, Spring 2007, vol. 32, no. 1, and a Sufi version in *Heart, Self and Soul: The Sufi Psychology of Growth, Balance, and Harmony* by Robert Frager (Quest Books, Wheaton, Illinois, 1999).

HEAVEN AND HELL

Books that include this story are: *One Hand Clapping: Zen Stories for all Ages*, by Martin Rafe (Rizzoli Publications, New York, 1995), *Doorways to the Soul, 52 Wisdom Tales From Around the World*, (The Pilgrim Press, Cleveland, Ohio, 1998), and *Soul Food, Stories to Nourish the Spirit and the Heart*, by Jack Kornfield and Christina Feldman, (Harper, San Francisco, 1991).

THE HEART THAT NO LONGER MOVES

I discovered this story in the Winter 2001, Volume 26, No. 4 issue of *Parabola* Magazine.

STANDING STILL

This story is attributed to Rabbi Levi Yitzhak of Berditchev; the story is found in *Tales of the Hasidim*, Martin Buber and Olga Marx, (Schocken Books, New York). One of the best books on the early Hasidic masters is *Souls on Fire: Portraits and Legends of Hasidic Masters by Elie Wiesel (Random House, New York, 1972)*. A Zen version can be found in *Soul Food, Stories to Nourish the Spirit and the Heart.*

CONEJITO AND THE WAX DOLL

This tale can be found in *Yaqui Myths and Legends*, by Ruth Warner Giddings (The University of Arizona Press, 1983) and *Cuento del Conejo y el Coyote* by Victor and Gloria De La Cruz (Circulo de Arte, Mexico City, 1998). This tale is similar to *Br'er Rabbit and the Tar Baby*, popular in the Southeastern United States. See *The Children's Hour, Myths and Legends* by Marjorie Barrows (Grolier Inc., New York, 1966).

THE LOTUS ON THE ROOF

Stuart Blackburn presents this story in *Moral Fictions, Tamil Folktales from Oral Tradition* (Suomalainen Tiedeakatemia Academia Scientiarum Fennica, Helsinki, 2001).

THE BROKEN MIRRORS

This story is also found in *Moral Fictions, Tamil Folktales from Oral Tradition*. It's similar to the moral the "don't count you chickens before they hatch" motif.

THE TWO WOLVES

I have heard this story many times, and it is widely available on the Internet; I have not found a written source. Friends at the Healing Story Alliance list serve pointed me to Wolf Song of Alaska at www.wolfsongalaska.org, listing the author as unknown.

THE CHERRY BLOSSOMS

I found this story in *One Hand Clapping: Zen Stories for all Ages*, and *Kindness: A Treasury of Buddhist Wisdom for Children and Parents*, by Sarah Conover (Eastern Washington University Press, 2001).

THE SPIRIT WHO LIVED IN A TREE

This story is said to be a Jataka tale, or a Buddha birth story; however, my research never turned it up as such. I found it in *New Junior Classics Myths and Legends*, vol. 3 (PF Collier & Son, 1952).

THE COLOR OF GOD

I first heard this story from the Self-Realization Fellowship lessons by Paramhansa Yogananda, which I took as a teenager. In *The Hero with a Thousand Faces* (MJF Books, New York, 1949), Joseph Campbell says that it's from the Yoruba tribe of Africa. It's also found in *Wisdom Tales From Around the World* by Heather Forest (August House Books, Little Rock, 1996).

CHILDREN OF WAX

That life is created out of something that has died is a familiar motif among many different agricultural societies. I found the Polynesian version, *Hina and the Eel* in the Winter 1998, Volume 23, No. 4, issue of *Parabola*, and the Tlingit story, *The Image That Came to Life* from the book, *Images of a People: Tlingit Myths and Legends*, by Mary Helen Pelton and Jacqueline DiGennaro (Libraries Unlimited, Inc., Englewood, Colorado, 1992). The version I am using comes from Alexander McCall Smith's book, *Children of Wax* (Interlink Publishing Group, Inc., Brooklyn, 1999).

THE DOVE AND THE SPARROW

I heard this story from my sister, Narada Dasi Johnson, when I was young. Later, working as a Spellbinder storyteller, I heard a Chinese version in which a bird is in position to hold up the sky if it falls. He says he is willing to do his part, even though he is only one tiny, little bird.

About the Author

Sydney Solis, RYT, has been bringing the joy and healing of yoga and stories to children and adults internationally since 2000. She is the author of *Storytime Yoga™: Teaching Yoga to Children Through Story*, which was nominated for the Anne Izard Storytellers' Choice Award. She is also the author of numerous audio recordings, which can be found on her website at www.StorytimeYoga.com.

Sydney has more than 350 hours in the Anusara Yoga tradition, and has trained with founder John Friend. She now studies Ashtanga at Richard Freeman's Yoga Workshop. She has taught English as a Second Language tutor in public elementary and high schools, and worked in her children's Montessori classrooms for seven years.

Sydney teaches her method of Storytime Yoga™ to teachers and parents in workshops internationally, calling for world peace in the name of children. An associate of the Joseph Campbell Foundation, she has produced three World Peace Interfaith Storytelling Gatherings.

She lives in a little house with a big garden with her husband, four children, two cats, and one dog in Boulder, Colorado.

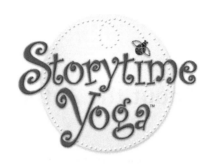

REORDER COUPON

To Reorder More copies of this book, please visit:
www.storytimeyoga.com

OTHER BOOKS, AUDIO AND VIDEO AVAILABLE:

BOOKS
Storytime Yoga™: Teaching Yoga to Children Through Story

AUDIO
The Peddler's Dream: Wisdom Stories from Around the World

MP3 Download Accompaniment to
Storytime Yoga™: Teaching Yoga to Children Through Story

DVD
The Peddler's Dream

VIDEO DOWNLOAD
The Peddler's Dream: Storytime Yoga Live

Stories of Faith, Healing and Transformation

Learn to use the Storytime Yoga™ method in depth.
Sign up for a Parent/Teacher training in your area
or for internet classes.

Sign up with the *Lotus*, The Free E-zine of Storytime Yoga™,
with Sydney's teaching schedule and free audio and story!

Join the League of Yogic Storytellers (LOYS).

The Mythic Yoga Studio, LLC
PO Box 3805
Boulder, CO 80307

NOTES:

NOTES:

CPSIA information can be obtained at www.ICGtesting.com
Printed in the USA
LVOW011433051012

301680LV00001B/36/P

9 780977 706310